ROUTLEDGE LIBRARY EDITIONS:
NURSE EDUCATION AND
NURSING CARE

Volume 18

INTERNATIONAL ISSUES IN NURSING RESEARCH

INTERNATIONAL ISSUES IN NURSING RESEARCH

Edited by
SHIRLEY M. STINSON
AND
JANET C. ROSS-KERR

Routledge
Taylor & Francis Group

LONDON AND NEW YORK

First published in Great Britain in 1986 by Croom Helm Ltd.

This edition first published in 2026
by Routledge
4 Park Square, Milton Park, Abingdon, Oxon OX14 4RN

and by Routledge
605 Third Avenue, New York, NY 10158

Routledge is an imprint of the Taylor & Francis Group, an informa business

British Library Cataloguing in Publication Data
A catalogue record for this book is available from the British Library

ISBN: 978-1-041-11658-5 (Set)
ISBN: 978-1-041-10677-7 (Volume 18) (hbk)
ISBN: 978-1-041-10680-7 (Volume 18) (pbk)
ISBN: 978-1-003-65631-9 (Volume 18) (ebk)

DOI: 10.4324/9781003656319

Publisher's Note
The publisher has gone to great lengths to ensure the quality of this reprint but points out that some imperfections in the original copies may be apparent.

Disclaimer
The publisher has made every effort to trace copyright holders and would welcome correspondence from those they have been unable to trace.

International Issues in Nursing Research

**Edited by
Shirley M. Stinson
and Janet C. Kerr**

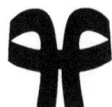

CROOM HELM
London & Sydney

© 1986 Shirley M. Stinson and Janet C. Kerr
Croom Helm Ltd, Provident House, Burrell Row,
Beckenham, Kent BR3 1AT

Croom Helm Australia Pty Ltd, Suite 4, 6th Floor,
64-76 Kippax Street, Surry Hills, NSW 2010, Australia

British Library Cataloguing in Publication Data

International issues in nursing research.
   1. Nursing — Research
   I. Stinson, Shirley M. II. Kerr, Janet C.
   610.73'072   RT81.5

   ISBN 0-7099-4437-3

and

The Charles Press, Publishers, PO Box 15715
Philadelphia, Pennsylvania 19103

Library of Congress Catalog Card Number
86-70460
ISBN 0-914783-11-4

Printed and bound in Great Britain
by Billing & Sons Limited, Worcester.

CONTENTS

Contents

Contents

TABLES AND FIGURES

iv

PREFACE

The impact of the first International Nursing Research Conference, held in Edinburgh, Scotland in 1981, was a powerful one. The need for discussion of various issues and problems on an international basis was a persuasive characteristic of that event. The discovery that many of the problems facing the profession in general and nurse researchers in particular are similar across different countries underscores the utility of nursing literature aimed at developing an international perspective. Such an approach contributes to wider awareness and better understanding of the central issues and problems, and lessens the tendency to reinvent the wheel.

Although there have been several international collections of research articles centered around a particular topic published to date, there has been no previous attempt to address matters of professional concern, including policy development, in the area of nursing research on an international basis. The present work, by no means exhaustive, represents an initial effort to provide a beginning perspective, and it is our hope that more such literature will be seen in the future.

Shirley M. Stinson, RN, EdD, LLD
Janet C. Kerr, RN, PhD

Shirley M. Stinson, RN, EdD, LLD

Dr. Stinson is a generalist, with experience in nursing practice, administration, teaching and research. She is Associate Dean for Graduate Education and Research Development at The University of Alberta, where she teaches in the Faculty of Nursing and in the Department of Health Services Administration and Community Medicine. She has consulted widely, both nationally and internationally. Dr. Stinson is a Past President of the Canadian Nurses Association.

Janet C. Kerr, RN, BScN, MS, PhD

Dr. Kerr is a Professor and Associate Dean (Undergraduate Education) at the Faculty of Nursing, University of Alberta. She has conducted research in the areas of quality assurance, geriatric needs and services and the financing of nursing education. She is a Past President of the Alberta Association of Registered Nurses and is interested in trends and issues in nursing, nursing of elderly people and research on the quality of nursing care. She has published many articles and is co-author of *Contemporary Issues in Canadian Law for Nurses*.

Chapter One

DESCRIPTIVE AND EXPERIMENTAL APPROACHES TO NURSING PROBLEMS: ISSUES IN DESIGN

Peggy Leatt

Empirical research has been by far the most common approach characterizing investigations into nursing practice to date.   Since empirical research involves the collection of information from the field, specifically from the persons under study, it seems logical that this approach would have been used with relative frequency to investigate a practice discipline such as nursing. In spite of its apparent popularity as an approach to nursing research, journals are prolific with discussions of problems and limitations in researchers' abilities to draw valid conclusions from many empirical studies.   Some of these difficulties seem to stem from researchers' limitations in formulating a specific design or approach suitable for the complex nursing research questions to be addressed.

RESEARCH DESIGN: PROCESS AND OUTCOME

One of the most creative aspects of research is to design the approach that will be employed to ensure that the research question being posed can be answered satisfactorily.   The specific design selected by the investigators will enable them to answer questions validly, objectively, accurately and economically (Kerlinger, 1973, p. 301).
        The term *research design* is used in two ways. First, as a process, research design involves planning, structuring and outlining strategies that the investigator will use to answer the research questions. Second, as an outcome, research design may be viewed as an end product comprising perhaps an elegant framework which will enable adequate testing of relationships among variables.

1

Research design has some crucial purposes. Its most important function is to structure investigation in such a way as to test the question at hand. The design should provide a map of the kinds and sequence of activities required to achieve the research objectives. Developing a detailed design early in the research process increases the probability of dealing effectively with unexpected problems and sticky issues which often occur as the research progresses.

According to Kerlinger (p. 100) research design has two fundamental purposes. The first purpose is to provide answers to research questions, while the second, more technical purpose, is to achieve control. In constructing appropriate designs, investigators attempt to achieve control in three different but interrelated ways. First, they wish to maximise the experimental variance. This means that the researcher attempts to design, plan and conduct research so that the experimental conditions are as different as possible. Second, the investigator wants to control extraneous variables, that is to be able to nullify the effects on dependent variables of any variables which are not directly related to the investigation. Third, the researcher tries to minimise or control any variability in measures which could have occurred by chance (pp. 306-313).

The selection of a research design is not normally a simple event which can be concluded hastily. Of course, any discussion of the design stems from the nature of the research question to be addressed. In all cases the design should be tailored to the individual problem inherent in the research; consequently, in reading research reports one rarely finds two investigations in which identical approaches have been used. Exceptions to this might occur when there is a deliberate attempt to replicate or duplicate a previous study.

Usually there is more than one person involved in deciding upon the most appropriate approach. This is particularly true in a practice discipline such as nursing where the design may be constrained by limitations imposed by the practical setting of the research. It is often helpful to discuss possible research designs with colleagues, practitioners, statisticians, and so on. If the design has the potential for being relatively complex, then expert consultation from someone with experience using the specific approach proposed may be necessary.

Since the evolution of scientific methods, there has been a tendency to imply that the most appropriate research design is always one modelled on the experimental method. Roberts (1974) and others have pointed out the importance of tailoring the research design to the specific research question and the nature of the phenomena under investigation. For example, Roberts maintains that while experimental methods may be most appropriate for investigating physical phenomena, the nature and conditions of the social sciences may be sufficiently different (even more complex) to warrant different kinds of research approaches. Part of the problem in the social sciences stems from the general lack of understanding of the complexities of human behavior and researchers' limitations in being able to conceptualise and design strategies which will provide valid additions to the body of existing knowledge.

But still there is a subconscious feeling amongst many researchers that "good" research has an experimental design and failure to use this approach implies a second rate investigation. This feeling can be particularly prevalent amongst researchers who come from a discipline or occupation which is just beginning to embark into the field of research. Greater contributions to knowledge may be made through a descriptive approach tailored to the individual problem rather than using experimental methods inappropriately. The most important factor is the requirement in all types of research to adhere to rigorous standards of scientific investigation and truthful recording of all events.

It seems clear that there is no one best method that can be applied irrespective of the research problem at hand. The most appropriate design will be contingent upon a variety of complex factors including the research question, the context of the research, the subjects to be involved, the level of knowledge and previous research in the area, accessibility of reliable and valid measurement instruments and the human resources available.

SOME TYPES OF RESEARCH DESIGNS

There is a tendency amongst researchers to classify approaches to research into two general categories, descriptive or experimental. Descriptive research usually aims to describe an event, phenomenon or situation and its main contribution lies in the precise definition of terms and accurate documentation (Clark & Hockey, 1979, p. 18). Experimental research occurs when investigators have full control over the situation and independent variables may be manipulated in order to observe their influence upon dependent variables. Usually in experimental research it is possible to use randomisation in order to identify more clearly cause and effect relationships.

The basic underlying difference between descriptive and experimental approaches therefore is the extent to which the investigator is able to exert control over the variables in the study. A number of researchers, however, have suggested that much empirical research may have both a descriptive and an experimental (or at minimum, analytic) component thus making it both difficult and somewhat arbitrary to classify the research into either the descriptive or experimental categories (Kajuzny & Veney, 1980, p. 50).

It would seem more realistic then to conceive of various approaches to research on a continuum of control. Clearly, laboratory experiments would be at the high end of the continuum in that the researcher has a high degree of control over the experimental situation. At the other extreme, descriptive, qualitative research would be placed at the low end of the continuum in that investigators generally have little control over events which have usually taken place previously and are often interpreted after they have occurred. The control continuum and approximate locations of some common types of research designs are illustrated in Figure 1.1. These types are *not* meant to be comprehensive of all possible research designs or in fact to be mutually exclusive. Dotted lines are used to indicate that boundaries between the types may be blurred in that an individual project could be ranked somewhere between types or as a combination of types.

The actual position of a particular research project in relation to this control continuum, however, has some implications for the kinds of activities which are feasible during the research and the generalisability of research findings. For example, in research at the lower end of the continuum there is likely to be greater difficulty in interpreting results. Findings are likely to be less generalisable and there will probably be a greater number of rival hypotheses which will

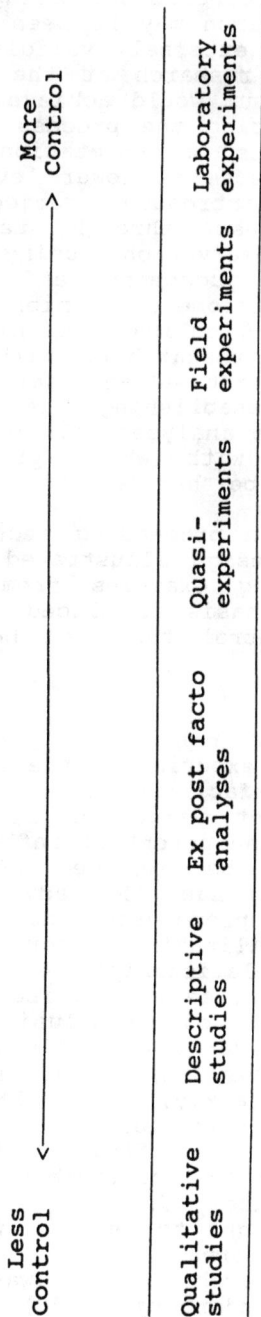

Figure 1.1

THE CONTINUUM OF CONTROL

Less Control

More Control >

| Qualitative studies | Descriptive studies | Ex post facto analyses | Quasi- experiments | Field experiments | Laboratory experiments |

hinder simple conclusions being drawn. In other words the research may be seen as lacking in both internal and external validity. It could be expected that research at the higher end of the control continuum would achieve a higher degree of objectivity during the process of the research as well as in the interpretation of findings. In contrast, projects at lower levels of control may deliberately introduce subjectivity into the research process through techniques such as participant observation, using practitioners' or other experts' judgements and providing researchers' and practitioners' opinions in the interpretations of the implications of results. It is probable that researchers with high control can conduct more precise analyses, that is the kind aimed at establishing relationships between variables. The analyses will be facilitated by the greater ease with which problems of internal validity can be handled in the more controlled situation.

During the proceeding sections the six types of research design illustrated in Figure 1.1 are discussed using examples from nursing research. Particular emphasis is placed upon the nature and degree of control that can be achieved by each approach.

Laboratory Experiments
In laboratory experiments the research is isolated in a physical facility where complete control over the independent variables in the study can be obtained and the potential influences of extraneous variables can be excluded (Kerlinger, p. 398). This approach has the advantage that greater precision of procedures and definitions can be achieved, facilitating later replication. Cause and effect relationships between independent and dependent variables can be isolated which can lead to more clear cut conclusions about findings. There are however some difficulties in attempting to use laboratory experiments for nursing practice research. Clearly, the laboratory situation creates an artificial environment for nursing research; thus any findings from the laboratory setting may not be replicable in the realities of nursing practice. In general, laboratory experiments are thought to be high in internal validity but weak in external validity.

The research of Kagawa-Busby, Heitkemper, Hanson and Vanderburg (1980) clearly illustrates the advantages and disadvantages of laboratory experiments. These investigators were interested in finding out what effects nasogastric tube feeding administered at different temperatures might have on gastric motility, total gastrointestinal transit time and diarrhoea and subjects' perceptions of adverse sensations and symptoms. Previous studies had implied that different temperatures of liquid diet feedings could affect both gastric responses and subjective sensations but findings had been inconclusive. Accordingly, the researchers undertook a laboratory experiment to evaluate the effects of feedings of different temperatures in a controlled situation.

The subjects were six paid volunteers, four females and two males, with no history of gastrointestinal surgery or pathology. The subjects came to the laboratory following an overnight fast. Each subject was positioned in bed with the head elevated 45 degrees and a nasogastric tube was introduced. The subjects were oriented to the laboratory setting and pretesting of one feeding procedure was completed before the experiment began. During the experiment subjects were given liquid diet feedings at three different temperatures: cold (8-11° C.); room (23-26° C.); and warm (body temperature, 36-39° C.). The participants were not told the actual temperature of each feeding. The effects of the experimental procedures were measured by changes in recordings of gastric motility, intragastric temperature, and subjective sensations. A total of 60 tube feedings was administered to the six subjects in feeding sessions of 10 trials. Total records were available for 109 hours of observation. The findings indicated that there was no relationship between temperature of feeding and gastric motility when this was assessed by amplitude and frequency of contractions and the time taken for digestive activity to occur. Some participants experienced abdominal cramping and diarrhoea between six to nine hours after receiving cold feedings. This reaction did not seem to occur following room temperature and warm feedings. These results, however, were confounded by the fact that one participant was menstruating so it is not known whether the abdominal cramps were attributable to this factor or the cold feeding. The study suggested that if refrigerated feeding is used it should be allowed to warm to room temperature or it should be administered slowly to allow the food to come to a warm temperature before it reaches the stomach.

The use of a laboratory experiment design for this research provided a number of advantages. Clearly, there was some highly specialised equipment necessary which may not have been easily used in the practice setting. But the main advantages of the approach relate to the benefits in controlling problems of internal validity. Campbell and Stanley (1963, p. 5), in their classic work, outlined factors which can jeopardise the internal validity of experiments. These include: history, maturation, testing, instrumentation, statistical regression, selection, experimental mortality and selection-maturation interaction. Through the laboratory context, the researchers were able to control possible effects of history and maturation. For example, because the subjects were located in an isolated situation there was a limited number of stimuli that they received apart from the experimental procedure. Maturation, for example, in terms of the rate of subjects' growing hungrier was controlled by the time intervals between feedings. The testing and instrumentation procedures were consistent across all participants and pretesting was carried out initially. In terms of the possibility of problems associated with the selection of participants such as selection bias, statistical regression and so on, these were minimal for this experiment because inclusion criteria indicated that the subjects were to be healthy, with no previous problems of a gastric or systemic nature.

Major weaknesses in the use of the laboratory experiment approach for this research relate to limitations in external validity. For example, the results in terms of adverse reactions to cold feedings could be different in non-experimental settings. It is possible that patients' reactions to cold feedings could be exacerbated because of other tensions and stresses experienced because of hospitalisation. Also, reactions to feeding temperature could be different when non-healthy subjects are examined, i.e. there may be different physiological reactions to feeding temperature when patients have pathological problems associated with the gastrointestinal tract. To overcome some of these limitations to external validity, it would be necessary to approach the research questions in terms of a field experiment. This kind of an approach would present other problems, for example, the accessibility of patients for this type of experiment and the ethics of conducting experiments of such intensity on patients who are ill.

Field Experiments

A field experiment is research conducted in a realistic situation where one or more independent variables are manipulated by the researcher to observe their effects. Usually, field experiments offer fewer possibilities for control than laboratory experiments (Kerlinger, p. 401). Field experiments have many advantages because they take place in real life settings where behaviors can be observed as they occur naturally. The underlying objective in field experiments is to control as much of the context of the research as possible so that the study will mirror the controlled conditions associated with laboratory situations as rigorously as feasible. Field experiments are also considered useful approaches for testing theories as well as examining practical problems.

Limitations to field experiments relate to the lack of ability in some settings to achieve sufficient control over the independent variable(s). This may be particularly true in clinical nursing studies where nursing care is so interdependent with services provided by other professionals. A second limitation to field experiments is the lack of feasibility in some research to use randomisation. This limits the extent to which extraneous variables can be controlled and thus the generalisability of findings.

Field experiments also require considerable expertise on the part of the researchers to solicit assistance from field agencies and to include them in the design of the approach. Interpersonal skills of this type are essential if the field experiment is to be accomplished without unnecessary intrusion into patient care.

The study of Goldberg and Fitzpatrick (1980) was designed as a field experiment to investigate whether nursing intervention in the form of movement therapy would improve levels of morale and self esteem within an aged institutionalised population. Basing their work on theories of aging and previous sociogerontological research, the investigators hypothesised that institutionalised aged individuals who participated in a movement therapy group would show significantly greater improvements in morale, loneliness, dissatisfaction and attitude towards their own aging than individuals who did not participate in a movement therapy group. A sample of 30 persons 65 years of age or older was selected from individuals residing in a 100-bed nursing home in a metropolitan area. Inclusion criteria were that persons had to be oriented to time, place and person; able to speak and understand English; able to complete morale and self esteem scales; and physically able to participate in a movement therapy group. Subjects were not screened on the basis of sex, length of time in institution or physical disabilities.

The experimental treatment consisted of 12 movement therapy sessions led by a professional nurse. The general goal of the treatment was to increase the range of verbal and non-verbal behavior of participants. The nurse's role was to encourage participation of individuals but no specific movement routines were taught or specific responses expected.

The sample of subjects was randomly divided into two groups with 15 members each thus allowing random assignment of individuals to the experimental and control groups for comparative purposes. The control group received no treatment apart from the activities scheduled routinely in the nursing home. Men and women were about equally divided between each group, there being more women than men.

Measures of the outcome variables (morale, loneliness and attitudes towards aging) were taken at times pre and post experimental treatment using a variety of scales which had been used in previous research and had demonstrated an acceptable degree of reliability and validity.

Since the experimental and control group had not been matched *a priori* on age, total disability and length of time in the institution, t-tests for differences in means between the two groups were examined. The results of this analysis showed individuals in the control group had been institutionalised for a significantly (0.05 level) longer period of time than individuals in the experimental group. Accordingly, analysis of covariance was computed on the post-test scores adjusting for initial differences in pretest scores and length of institutionalisation. The findings indicated that individuals who participated in the movement therapy group demonstrated greater improvement in total morale and attitudes towards their own aging than the individuals in the control group. There was also a tendency for individuals in the movement therapy group to show greater self-esteem but there were no differences between the two groups on measures of loneliness or agitation (interpreted as an aspect of morale).

The researchers were able to draw connections between their findings and the larger knowledge of social gerontology. In addition, they concluded that skilled nursing intervention could play an important role in improving levels of morale and attitudes towards their own aging of institutionalised aged individuals.

The approach used by Goldberg and Fitzpatrick is an illustration of one of Campbell and Stanley's (p. 13) true experimental designs. This design, the pretest-post-test control group design, is not considered to be the strongest true experimental design but it is an approach which facilitates control of the seven threats to internal validity mentioned earlier. For example, effects of history are controlled by obtaining pre and post-test scores for both experimental and control groups in that intervening historical events would probably occur for both groups. The approach attempts to control for equivalence in maturation and testing effects since these also should be equal for both groups. Selection factors were not totally ruled out in this case since there was not full assurance that individuals assigned to the experimental treatment were equivalent on all variables. This inequivalence, specifically that control group subjects had been institutionalised significantly longer than those in the experimental group, was an important issue which required a particular kind of statistical strategy to clarify whether or not improvements in the experimental group's morale and attitudes towards their own aging could be attributed to the experimental treatment or whether it was an artifact of their having been in the institution for a shorter length of time. The researchers employed analysis of covariance, a technique suggested by Campbell and Stanley (p. 23), to show that the covariate, time in institution, consistently decreased the level of significant differences between the two groups on post-test scores. In terms of overall contribution to knowledge and understanding of the research question originally posed, this was an important finding.

From the results of this study, it was implied that nursing interventions in the form of group movement therapy would seem more likely to increase morale and improve attitudes towards aging when participants have been institutionalised for a shorter period of time. Clearly, these are critical factors to be considered in the design of further research in this area.

In terms of external validity, field experiments are generally stronger than laboratory experiments. The generalisability of findings in this instance may, however, have limitations for a number of reasons. First, the experiment was conducted in one institution and there may be unique characteristics of this nursing home which would preclude replication of the study. Second, the experimental treatment, i.e. exactly what was done in the group session, was left to the discretion of the individual nurse. Unless there are detailed records of procedures and full documentation of the independent variable in field experiments, they are difficult, if not impossible, to reproduce in other settings. Third, the participants themselves may not be representative of institutionalised aged persons. The sample size was small, and the inclusion criteria specific. Participants were not randomly selected from a larger population. Finally, as the researchers themselves suggest, it is not known whether participants in the experimental group scored better on the outcome measures than the control group because of the Hawthorne effect. Goldberg and Fitzpatrick recommend that future study designs should include another control group which receives some attention in order to control for possible Hawthorne effect.

Quasi-Experiments
Quasi-experiments occur, usually in field settings, when researchers are unable to achieve full control over the independent variables and/or are unable to use randomisation. According to Campbell and Stanley (p. 34), in quasi-experimental situations it is extremely important that the researcher be aware of the aspects of the experiment over which he/she does not have full control. Recognising that it is impossible to obtain an optimum level of control, with this approach the researcher should try to find the most suitable context for the study where there are the best opportunities for control. Clearly, with quasi-experiments there is a greater possibility of jeopardising the internal validity of the research and there may be considerable limitations on the generalisability of findings to other settings.

Quasi-experiments may take on several possible forms. For example, Campbell and Stanley (pp.

34-61) use the term to refer to single group experiments, nonequivalent control group designs, separate-sample pretest post-test designs, and so on. Another example of quasi-experiments is that of time-series analysis.

The time-series design is an approach in which successive measurements are taken of one or more groups and an experimental change is introduced at some period during the time series. An illustration of the principles of this type of research in nursing is the investigation of Edwards (1980) on changing breast self-examination behavior. The research question posed by Edwards was concerned with the relative effectiveness of various methods of breast self-examination education. In particular, she was interested in finding out whether certain types of educational programs were more likely than others to result in prolonged practice of self-examination after the initial instruction. Accordingly, the research approach needed to incorporate measurement of variables at several time periods before and after the implementation of the breast self-examination education program. Atypical of most quasi-experiments, the investigator was able to use randomisation. Fourteen field study sites were randomly selected from 24 available clinics in the region.

Four types of educational programs were developed: these were defined as modelling, guided practice, self-monitoring, and peer support. Modelling was considered as a control program since it was given to all groups as a base program. The other three programs were experimental and participants received supplementary programs. It was hypothesised that the experimental groups would show greater improvement between pre and post clinic practice of breast self-examination, would show greater knowledge of breast self-examination, and would have greater confidence in their ability to discover breast problems. It was also hypothesised that over the long term, the experimental groups would maintain a higher frequency of breast self-examination than the control group.

The total number of subjects in the study was 130. Inclusion criteria were that the woman should be a first time attender at the clinic, and should have indicated that she usually, sometimes, or never performed breast self-examination on initial questioning. Participants were randomly assigned to control and experimental programs. Data were collected at four time periods: before the educational program, that is at clinic registration;

immediately following the educational program; three months post clinic attendance; and six months post clinic attendance. Initial data analysis was performed on the demographic characteristics of the participants and no significant differences were found between the four groups in terms of mean income, education, age and minority status. Also, the subjects in the study were compared with the population of all the women who attended the 24 clinics and the participants were found to be representative of the larger population. There were no significant differences between the experimental and control groups in the pretest phase in the frequency with which participants indicated that they practised breast self-examination. These findings indicated that the groups were equivalent before the programs were administered. It is not essential in this discussion to explain the details of the four methods of education of breast self-examination; however, these were defined in detail and attempts were made to ensure that they were implemented consistently.

A Breast Self-Examination Knowledge and Practice Inventory was developed to use in the post-test period to evaluate the subjects' level of knowledge, ability to practise self-examination, and level of confidence in detecting breast abnormalities. This inventory was mailed to a random sample of one half of the subjects in the control and experimental groups three months after attendance at the clinic and to the remainder of the sample six months after attendance at the clinic. Overall, knowledge data was obtained for 60 percent of the sample, and breast self-examination behavior data for 85 percent of the sample.

The main finding was that education by modelling alone was just as effective in changing breast self-examination behavior as the other more extensive educational programs. This conclusion was drawn on the basis of no significant differences on post-test measures of subjects' level of knowledge, ability to practice self-examination, and level of confidence in detecting problems. When the frequency of breast self-examination over the long term was examined some interesting findings emerged. The frequency of self-examination increased for all groups over time with the control group being consistently lowest in all the follow-up time periods. After three months, the group which had been given education by modelling and guided practice had the highest mean frequency of breast self-examination. After six months, the group which had been given education by modelling and were also asked specifically to record and monitor their frequency of breast self-examination scored highest. These results raised some interesting issues concerning which factors are likely to influence over the long term, the extent to which women practise breast self-examination. Closer examination of the data from this study showed that, the overall frequency of self-examination had begun to decline across all groups between three to six months after the educational program.

Although the research of Edwards did not represent the classical time-series design because of the use of both control and experimental groups, the longitudinal design of the research is illustrative of some of the issues in multi-time period research. For example, one of the main problems of internal validity with this approach is one of history effects. Because the experiment takes place over a longer time period, it is not known whether different results would have been achieved if the experiment had taken place at a different point in time. For example, in the case of Edwards' research, had there been concurrent cancer campaigns which could have reached the full sample of participants and raised their awareness about the possibility of breast cancer, this could have influenced the decision to attend the clinic in the first place. Also, it is not known what other events may have taken place following the educational programs which could have influenced the subjects' tendencies to practise self-examination during the six month follow-up. For example, even events such as seasons, vacation time, weather, and so on, could potentially influence tendencies to carry out breast self-examination.

Usually internal validity problems of testing and instrumentation are not major factors with the time-series design; however, in Edwards' research it is interesting that the self-recording/monitoring group performed better over the long-term than the other groups. It is not known whether this approach may have produced certain biases. In terms of external validity, Campbell and Stanley (p. 42) warn researchers that a single experiment is never conclusive and it may be necessary to repeat the time-series analysis in other settings before a principle can be established. Clearly, there are still some questions and new hypotheses to be tested regarding the factors influencing women's likelihood of practising breast self-examination over the long term. Nevertheless, one of the strengths of Edwards' research was the thoroughness of steps taken to ensure that the sample of participants was representative of women attending the 24 clinics. Other researchers could attempt to replicate these findings with samples of both healthy women and those with breast abnormalities.

Ex Post Facto Analyses

In *ex post facto* analyses, there is no direct control over the independent variables because these are factors which already exist or events which have taken place in an earlier time (Campbell & Stanley, p. 70; Kerlinger, p. 378). It is research which takes place "after the fact". Examples of such independent variables are a person's intelligence, perceptions, personality, and so on. In *ex post facto* analyses inferences can be made about relationships amongst variables but it is difficult to establish causation. According to Kerlinger (p. 380), the basic logic underlying *ex post facto* analysis and experimentation is the same. The researcher wishes to establish the empirical validity of a conditional statement, that is, if p then q. Because the researcher does not control p (the independent variables) in *ex post facto* analysis, the establishment of validity of the conditional statement is more difficult. In addition, it is not possible to use randomisation as a mechanism of increasing control over extraneous variables, since the events have already occurred.

The main advantage of *ex post facto* analysis is its usefulness for investigating problems which are not amenable to experimentation. Some researchers may argue that some of the more interesting and exciting contributions in the behavioral sciences have been made through this approach because it is more suited than experimental methods to the true nature of social phenomena. An example of nursing research using this approach is the investigation of Papa (1980) of predictors of suicide intent in adults. Specifically, the objective in this research was to find out if there were relationships between a range of complex attitudes, hypothesised as independent variables, and the degree of suicide intent of suicide attempters, as the dependent variable. The independent variables included measures of suicide attempters' feelings of stress from life events, their feelings of hopelessness, their preferences

for inclusion and affection, and their preferences
for control and beliefs about locus of control.

The subjects consisted of 60 consecutive
suicide attempters entering a hospital for treatment following a suicide attempt. The subjects
were initially interviewed in the emergency room of
the hospital or on the medical units on admission.
A series of scales was administered to each
subject, completed in the presence of the investigator. The scales were measures of independent and
dependent variables, with previously established
levels of reliability and validity.

Background information on subjects' age, sex,
religion, marital status, number of marriages,
number of divorces, education, residence, number of
brothers and sisters, birth order and parents'
history was obtained. On analysis, the subjects
were found to be mostly female (68%), above 32
years of age (68%), with at least high school
education (79%) and had lived in their current
residence for less than one year (58%). In order
to test the relative importance of the independent
variables as predictors of the degree of suicide
intent of the suicide attempters, stepwise regression procedures were used. When all ten independent variables were used, 51% of the variance in
suicide intent could be accounted for.

The most important predictor of suicide intent
was the subjects' feelings of hopelessness. This
supported previous research findings. The other
independent variables did not emerge from the
analysis as strong predictors of suicide intent.
For example, it was expected that perceived stress
from life events, particularly for the six month
period prior to the suicide attempt, would be an
important predictor, yet the findings from the
multiple regression did not clearly demonstrate
this. In fact, from the order of the variables
entering the stepwise equation, perceived stress
from life events over the previous two years seemed
to be a more important factor than stress during
the previous six months. Such ambiguity in
interpretation of findings is typical in *ex post
facto* analyses where there has been no possibility
of manipulating the independent variables or in
using randomisation to control extraneous variables. Papa clearly points out in her research
report the limitations experienced in obtaining
reliable measures of some of the independent
variables and some of the alternative explanations
of the results. Stepwise regression can produce
problems in interpretation when there are

relationships among the independent variables. Such relationships tend to make the ordering and significance of variables entering the regression equation unstable and, therefore, difficult to interpret. There may be other predictors of levels of suicide intent in suicide attempters which were not taken into consideration in this investigation and Papa attempts to outline these in preparation for further research.

Descriptive Studies

As indicated earlier, descriptive studies have the objective of painting a picture of the real world through describing key characteristics of a situation. One of the main contributions of descriptive studies lies in the precise attention to accurate definitions of terms and documentation of events. Descriptive studies may consist of large surveys where typically a few select variables are measured across a large number of subjects. Probability sampling techniques are often employed so that a survey of a representative sample of the population is made. On the other hand, a descriptive study may consist of a case study of a single case with in depth description and documentation of a comprehensive range of variables.

Smith (1981) used a descriptive approach to explore the quality of working life of nurses working in a Health Maintenance Organisation (HMO). Since HMOs are a relatively new alternative to traditional services aimed primarily at reducing health care costs, it was considered important to find out the quality of the work environment provided for nurses in these settings. Based on previous literature on organisational behavior, Smith defined quality of working life as the extent to which organisational members thought they were able to satisfy their needs through their work experiences. Quality of working life was operationalised in terms of nurses' perceived job satisfaction, job tension and organisational commitment.

The participants in this study were 111 nurses employed in a single HMO. Three categories of nurses were included: licensed vocational nurses, registered nurses, and nurse practitioners. Each nurse was asked to complete a questionnaire which was returned to the investigator by mail. The questionnaire contained questions on personal characteristics (sex, age, number of dependents, level of education and number of years employed at the HMO), and the quality of working life variables. These were measured using scales from previous organisational studies. Data were analysed so that comparisons between the three categories of nurses could be made in terms of their perceptions of quality of working life in the HMO. Briefly, the results indicated that the nurse practitioners showed higher job satisfaction and organisational commitment than the registered nurses and licensed vocational nurses. This finding was in keeping with previous empirical research on the meaning of work to non-professional and semi-professional groups. Overall, the nurses' perceptions of the quality of their work life was that it was acceptable but not remarkable. None of the personal characteristics of the nurses appeared to be related to their perceptions of their work environment.

The advantage of the descriptive approach in this study was that it allowed detailed definition of aspects of quality of working life in the HMO. Since HMOs and the current emphasis in organisations on the concept of quality of working life are both relatively new phenomena, the descriptive approach was most appropriate. An obvious limitation to the research is its lack of external validity. It is not known whether nurses employed in other HMOs are likely to have similar perceptions of their quality of working life as the nurses employed in the HMO in this case study.

Qualitative Studies
The idea of qualitative research is not new. In the late 1930's there was a considerable interest in the use of qualitative techniques in the behavioral sciences. The main purpose for conducting qualitative research at that time was to find out details about issues or problems which would support the mainstream of research of that period in quantitative areas. In this early period qualitative research was generally thought to be sufficiently theoretical in nature and too impressionistic (Glaser & Strauss, 1967, p. 15). More recently, however, qualitative research has been gaining both popularity and credibility in the social sciences as a valuable research technique in its own right (see for examples: Jacobs, 1979; Agar, 1980). Qualitative studies are now being done to obtain more comprehensive understanding of natural phenomena as they occur in real life and in order to generate new theories.

The most important factor in qualitative research is the ability to assemble accurate evidence about phenomena. As Glaser and Strauss (pp. 17-18) point out, qualitative data may be used for both verification and testing of theories; quantitative and qualitative data are complementary and both may be necessary in attempting to answer some research questions. Qualitative research is essentially a process whereby the researcher observes phenomena of interest in the real world and then systematically assembles, assesses and analyses the observations. The process is often reiterative and incremental within the same study, the researcher needing to return to the field site for further data in order to answer the research questions.

Clearly, qualitative studies are most useful when the research question is exploratory and the main objective of the research is to broaden the general understanding of the situation or phenomenon. The process of this type of research demands particular kinds of skills from the researcher. Since most of the data are typically gathered through interviewing or observing, or involve participant observation techniques, human relation skills and knowledge of group dynamics are very important. The analysis of qualitative data may be through verbal accounts of events (often *verbatim*) or in some instances by quantifying the data through techniques such as content analysis. The interpretation of the findings and the modes of presentation are critical parts of the qualitative research process. The main advantages of qualitative research are the opportunities for detailed description of phenomena and events which lead to clarification of definitions and concepts, and the evolution of theories.

In health care, qualitative research is being used in situations where there are complex interactions amongst individuals, for example amongst patients, families and health care workers, and where behavior as a reflection of attitudes is an important issue (see for examples: Davis, 1980; Krulik, 1980). These relatively complex phenomena do not lend themselves easily to quantification. The main weaknesses relate to the extent to which the qualitative findings are reliable and, therefore, generalisable. Given the detailed observation, analysis, and needs for repeated observation and analysis in quantitative research, it is typically not possible to investigate a large number of phenomena, events or time phases within one study.

An example of a qualitative approach in nursing research is the investigation of Anderson (1981) who was interested in increasing the understanding of how parents construct social reality for a child with chronic illness. The focus in the research was on exploring how the parents conceptualised and described their child's illness and how they interacted with their child concerning the sickness. In reporting the investigation Anderson begins by setting the context for the research by describing the importance of culture to the social construction of illness and the role of the family in times of sickness.

Qualitative data were collected from four families whose chronically ill children ranged from 3 to 12 years of age. The chronically ill children had been diagnosed with long term medical problems and were being managed by their parents with support from health professionals in their own homes. Participant observation techniques were used to obtain parents' accounts of their child's illness and their management of it. Also, three visits, totalling 10-15 hours, were made to each family. Data were also collected from 12 families with well children for comparative purposes.

Anderson discusses the findings from her observations in terms of three main concepts: normalisation; lifestyle adjustments; and social interactions. In terms of the phenomenon of normalisation, Anderson describes parents' attempts to treat their child as normal in spite of their recognition of the child's chronic illness as being a pathological process. Parents who presented themselves as coping well with their situation interpreted this as meaning they were able to manage their circumstances as if they were not different from normal. In terms of lifestyle adjustments, the parents gave examples of a number of modifications which had been made to activities of daily living of family members so that the chronically ill child did not stand out as being different. Anderson used many *verbatim* quotes from her interviews with parents to describe these adjustments. Social interactions between the mother and child tended to be intensified because of the child's chronic illness and the need for someone in the family to assume a caretaker role. The sick children appeared to be somewhat isolated from their peers because of the limitations of their illness. They had few friends their age and tended to interact well with adults. Anderson draws some conclusions from her observations concerning the implications for nursing practice in terms of how nurses may help families to cope with a child's chronic illness. This qualitative approach was an appropriate one given the exploratory nature of the research and the limitations of previous knowledge about how parents respond to and cope with a child's chronic illness. Clearly, Anderson was able to gain considerable insight into how the families perceived the child's illness and their daily adaptations to it. The data were rich with examples obtained from the many hours of observation and interaction with the families. As with other qualitative studies, Anderson's findings may be limited in reliability and their generalisability to other families with children who are chronically ill.

SOME ADDITIONAL CONSIDERATIONS IN SELECTING DESIGNS FOR NURSING RESEARCH

Even though the most important criterion for the selection of an approach to research is that it must be appropriate to the research question, investigators still have some flexibility in choosing a design. Because of the practical nature of nursing, there are some additional factors which should be considered.

Nursing Research as Evaluation Research

A large number of the questions of interest in nursing research have to do with the effectiveness of nursing interventions or nursing programs. The main objective in this type of research is to provide information which will be useful for policy-making about nursing and for nursing care. Accordingly, this type of nursing research is fraught with similar challenges and problems as evaluation research conducted in other fields (see for example Overton and Stinson, 1977; Woody, 1980). Rossi and Berk (1981) have recently pointed out that the design of evaluation research should take into consideration the stage a program is at in its life history. For example, investigators may raise different questions about the efficacy of a program early in its life when the program is being designed, later when the program is being implemented and even later when the program has been in operation for some time. The first stage involves deciding what the program should be like. If the example of a program for post-myocardial infarction patients is used, the nursing research question might relate to identifying the needs of such patients in terms of exercise, diet, and social-psychological support. Once the program is designed, then nurse researchers might wish to explore the various means by which this type of program might be implemented and in which contexts. Later, the nursing research questions might relate to the extent to which the new post-myocardial infarction program was successful in terms of patient outcome measures.

Clearly these stages of the nursing program history would call for different research designs. During the needs assessment period, for example, qualitative exploratory approaches might be used to describe the needs as perceived by post-myocardial infarction patients themselves. When mechanisms for implementation of the program are being explored then a type of action or formative research would be appropriate. At the later stage when the effectiveness of the program is being evaluated then an experimental or quasi-experimental design would probably be most suitable. Given that the evaluation at any of these stages would take place under the constraints of practice settings, Rossi and Berk (p. 290) indicate that the design may be less than ideal, making the attention to technical concerns of the research all the more important.

Use of Theories in Nursing Research
Nursing research, like nursing practice, can draw upon theories from within nursing and from a wide range of other professional as well as academic disciplines. Some common examples include sociology, psychology, biology, physiology, and so on. The incorporation of theory into research has a number of advantages. First, it can provide a systematic framework for conceptualising the events that take place. Second, it can facilitate description of phenomena, and enable explanation and prediction of events. Third, theory can provide a practical guide to the collection and analysis of data during the research and writing up the research report. Fourth, the incorporation of theory in research can facilitate the enlargement of a body of knowledge through empirically testing aspects of the theory (for example see Glaser and Strauss, p. 3).

As with the choice of research design, the choice of theory in nursing research will depend upon the phenomena to be investigated. The inappropriate choice of theory may not only lead to invalid conclusions but may prevent the discovery of important findings and contributions to knowledge. Theory-based research in nursing is likely to become more common as theories of nursing practice evolve. Obviously, empirical research has a large role to play in both the development and validation of new theories of nursing.

The Nursing Practice Setting

The nursing practice settings have some relatively unique characteristics which need careful consideration in nursing research design. Since the underlying objective in most research design is to achieve as high a level of control as feasible, the nurse researcher will wish to monitor the practice setting as closely as possible. First the researcher will wish to design the study to ensure that the conditions inherent in the research (e.g. the program) are the same for all participants (see for example, Polit and Hungler, 1978). This may be difficult, for example, in an inpatient setting where there are multiple health team members with access to patients who come and go according to their own schedules. It may be especially difficult in nursing research to be able to design investigations so that the influence of a specific clinical nursing program on patients can be isolated from the influences of families, physicians and other health team workers. Second, the researcher will wish to ensure that the conditions of nursing interventions occur in the same time frame for all participants. For example, this may involve ensuring that data collection takes place at the same time of day, time of year or time after surgery, for each patient. A third problem with control in nursing practice settings is concerned with the units of analysis of interest. It may be desirable to design the research to obtain data from various sources, for example patients, family members, nurses, doctors, nursing records, unit records and hospital documents. It is important in the research design to ensure that there is consistency in the units of analysis so that comparability of data from different sources can be achieved.

Human Rights
Finally, any nursing research design must take into
consideration the rights of all human subjects who
are going to be involved. These may include
patients and staff directly included in the
research as well as those less directly involved
such as families, and administrative staff in the
hospital. There are various ways in which the
rights of individuals are taken into consideration
(Canadian Nurses Association, 1983; Diers, 1979;
Storch, 1982). Probably one of the first steps in
the design process in relation to human rights is
to develop a protocol for obtaining informed
consent from participants. Informed consent means
that each individual is provided with an explanation of the project as well as the risks and
benefits which might result from participation. A
second but related mechanism is to elaborate upon
how the individual's rights to privacy and confidentiality will be maintained. The procedures
involved here may be extensive, depending upon
whether it is necessary during data analysis to be
able to link specific responses to individual
participants. The third formal way in which there
is a check on the possibility of infringement of
the rights of individuals in nursing research is
through institutional reviews. Most universities
require research proposals to pass through an
internal review process. In addition, most health
agencies now have research committees which review
all research proposals from investigators wishing
to conduct research in their facility (see for
example Robb, 1981). It is clear, however, that
following these formal procedures is not sufficient
in itself to ensure human rights are protected;
nurse researchers and practitioners must be
constantly attuned to any possibility of infringement of human rights in research.

REFERENCES

Agar, M.H. (1980). *The professional stranger: An
informal introduction to ethnography.* New
York: Academic Press.

Anderson, J.M. (1981). The social construction of
illness experience: Families with a chronically-ill child. *Journal of Advanced Nursing, 6,*
427-434.

Campbell, D.T., & Stanley, J.C. (1963). *Experimental and quasi-experimental designs.* Chicago: Rand McNally, College Publishing Co.

Canadian Nurses Association. (1983). *Ethical guidelines for nursing research involving human subjects.* Ottawa: Author.

Clark, J.M., & Hockey, L. (1979). *Research for nursing: A guide for the enquiring nurse.* Aylesbury: HM & M Publishers.

Davis, A.J. (1980). Disability, home care and the caretaking role in the family. *Journal of Advanced Nursing, 5,* 475-484.

Diers, D. (1979). *Research in nursing practice.* Toronto: J.B. Lippincott.

Edwards, V. (1980). Changing breast self-examination behaviour. *Nursing Research, 29,* 301-306.

Glaser, B.S., & Strauss, A.L. (1967). *The discovery of grounded theory: Strategies for qualitative research.* Chicago: Aldine Publishing Co.

Goldberg, W.G., & Fitzpatrick, J.J. (1980). Movement therapy with the aged. *Nursing Research, 29,* 339-346.

Jacobs, J. (1979). *Qualitative sociology: A method to madness.* New York: The Free Press.

Kagawa-Busby, K.S., Heitkamper, B.C., Hanson, R.L., & Vanderburg, V.V. (1980). Effects of diet temperature or tolerance of enteral feedings. *Nursing Research, 29,* 276-280.

Kajuzny, A.D., & Veney, J.E. (1980). *Health service organisations: A guide to research and assessment.* Berkeley: McCutchan Publishing Corp.

Kerlinger, F.N. (1973). *Foundations of behavioral research* (2nd ed.). Toronto: Holt, Rinehart & Winston, Inc.

Krulik, T. (1980). Successful 'normalizing' tactics of parents of chronically-ill children. *Journal of Advanced Nursing, 5,* 573-578.

Overton, P., & Stinson, S.M. (1977). Program evaluation in health services: The use of experimental designs. *Journal of Advanced Nursing, 2,* 137-146.

Papa, L.L. (1980). Response to life events as predictors of suicidal behavior. *Nursing Research, 29,* 362-370.

Polit, D., & Hungler, B. (1978). *Nursing research: Principles and methods.* Toronto: J.B. Lippincott.

Robb, S.S. (1981). Nurse involvement in institutional review boards: The service setting perspective. *Nursing Research, 30,* 27-29.

Roberts, M.J. (1974). On the nature and conditions of the social sciences. *Daedalus, 103,* 47-64.

Rossi, P.H., & Berk, R.A. (1981). An overview of evaluation strategies and procedures. *Human Organisation, 40,* 287-299.

Smith, H.L. (1981). Nurses' quality of working life an a HMO: A comparative study. *Nursing Research, 30,* 54-58.

Storch, J. (1982). *Patients' rights: Ethical and legal issues in health care and nursing.* Toronto: McGraw-Hill Ryerson Limited.

Woody, M.F. (1980). An evaluator's perspective. *Nursing Research, 29,* 74-79.

Chapter Two

HISTORICAL NURSING RESEARCH

Janet C. Kerr

Civilisations have long placed much value on the transmission of cultural folklore from one genera-tion to another. This was as true of the ancient world as it is of many cultures which exist today. Even in the Western world currently, there would appear to be growing emphasis placed on reporting and recording of descriptions of important events, practices and people in the society as well as the preservation of such records. In North America the striking growth and development of local historical societies along with the concomitant phenomenon of the search for one's familial 'roots', serve as illustrations of the increasing value placed on historical endeavours at the community level in the midst of the fast pace of life in the modern world.
 In looking for reasons to explain why impor-tance is placed on knowing about and preserving information from events occurring in the past, one needs to look no further than the value to be found in its perceived usefulness to society. It has been said that: 'What memory is to the individual, history is to the human race' (Hayes & Moon, 1929, p. 1). Margaret Mead commented with regret on loss of information about civilisations and cultures:

> When those of us who are now middle-aged or old were children, we read in the history books romantic tales of lost arts, and our imagina-tions were caught first by tales of lost meth-ods of tempering steel or making stained glass, later by the realisation that there were whole civilisations which were lost, in that to-day no single man or woman can carry in his gait and bearing, in his speech and way of living, the intricate pattern that had been Greece or Persia, Egypt or ancient Peru (1955, p. 19).

Just as the ancient Babylonians believed it important to record information about their culture in
the form of hieroglyphics on clay tablets, so too
in the modern world increasing emphasis is being
placed upon developing ways of recording, storing
and preserving data so that future generations will
not experience difficulty in gaining access to it.
Exemplifying such an attitude and at the same time
attempting to teach children to value history,
local schools often have projects to develop 'time
capsules', these being containers of carefully
collected and preserved information, stored for
disclosure to a new generation of citizens at a
specified future date. The purpose of such an
undertaking is to enclose written materials and
objects which will give teachers and students 50 or
100 years later a 'bird's eye view' of living and
education at the present time. It is thus widely
accepted that the lessons to be learned from history are believed to be important in order to assist
in the understanding of contemporary society and in
developing approaches to meet the challenges of
today as well as those of the future.

**RELEVANCE OF HISTORICAL RESEARCH IN PROFESSIONAL
DISCIPLINES**

In a professional discipline where practice is a
fundamental and important component, the associated
responsibilities for research and scholarship are
widely believed to be vital to developing and
improving practice. Although there is considerable
dispute about whether or not this is actually true
at this point in the development of the profession,
some effort would appear to be directed toward the
achievement of such a goal. Shaver (1978) notes
that the scope of knowledge required in nursing
with its scientific and humanitarian aspects underscores 'the need for philosophical and historical
scholars in nursing who can ask crucial questions
from the perspective of nursing' (p. 115). If
there is not substantial commitment within the
profession to examining theoretical and clinical
problems from a variety of perspectives, discipli-
nary development will be hindered and held back.
    It is well known that the need for philosophi-
cal as well as historical methods of inquiry to
approach problems and questions which arise in a
discipline is well-accepted in such professions as
law and medicine where there has always been considerable attention paid to history. In nursing,

however, where research is yet in its infancy and there is a dearth of individuals qualified to conduct investigations, even fewer are prepared to address historical questions. Perhaps this circumstance is rooted in so much emphasis being placed upon preparing researchers to undertake highly quantitative and scientific experiments in clinical nursing practice, that the need to encourage those with a bent for things historical to develop expertise in historical research methods has been overlooked. In a study of Canadian accomplishments in research and scholarship, Professor Symons has observed that:

> Little has been written about the history and achievements of the profession in Canada. There have been almost no biographical studies of outstanding members of the profession. It is regrettable that some of the leaders in Canadian nursing seem to have received more recognition in the United States, and in Britain and Western Europe, than in their own country (p. 212).

Historical research in nursing is needed to provide knowledge and understanding of the achievements of and contributions to the profession as well as to the larger society by individual nurses and groups of nurses and about significant events and forces which have shaped the character of the profession. The essence of nursing and the nature of the professional identity will be more readily understood as a result of studies which are undertaken within such contexts. For those entering the profession, learning about the achievements of nursing leaders and the progress of the profession over time can provide a basis for professional socialization as well as encouraging new initiatives in desired directions, but the history of nursing is a factor which should enter into the perspective of every nurse, and at all career stages.

Ashley has criticised the historical work which has been undertaken thus far: 'Historical research in nursing has, to date, consisted of purely descriptive reporting of data without any conceptual analysis of their meaning for nurses and for society' (1978, p. 29). She further decries the absence of references to documents outside the field to allow for better understanding of the meaning of professional events in the context of the larger society. The more serious allegation

that 'much of the written history of nursing has
been used to support illusions that foster false
pride' (p. 29) would unfortunately appear to be
fair comment on much historical work in the profession to date. Ashley asserts that the reason for
this sorry plight may be found in the following:

Within nursing, devaluation of our history is
the direct cause of not having any authentic
historical studies to give us knowledge to use
in deepening the conscience of our humanity.
Our identity has suffered greatly because we
have not carefully studied our history and
incorporated historical knowledge into theoretical and clinical teachings. Without this
knowledge, the foundations of nursing scholarship and practice have indeed been shaky (p.
29).

ISSUES IN HISTORICAL RESEARCH METHODS

The range of problems which may be addressed
through historical methods is considerable. One
may wish to reconstruct and/or describe past
events, to present an analysis which may serve to
explain situations and relationships or to create
an integrated and meaningful narrative of occurrences in the recent or more distant past. Thus
one may choose to study the life and work of a
noteworthy nursing leader or the origins and development over time of a health care agency, a professional organisation or a school of nursing. In
studying topics which are as broad as the foregoing, the researcher must necessarily address questions of art, philosophy, ethics, science as well
as those which relate to other disciplines. However, as has been noted above, approaches to nursing
questions of an historical nature should avoid the
insular and self-serving stance of the profession
alone, and need to consider the issues in relation
to society as a whole.

There are important methodological differences
between historical and other kinds of research such
as experimental, quasi-experimental and survey
research. The data in historical research cannot
really be generated except in the memories of those
who were party or witness to events under study.
The events themselves cannot be repeated or manipulated, only considered, examined, discussed and
compared with other occurrences. Unfortunately,
one cannot turn the clock back for first-hand

observation and control of the situation. To study history is to study the past with all the inherent problems and difficulties which that entails. It is not possible to observe directly, to manipulate, to control or to replicate, principles fundamental to the experimental method. Although description is commonly a purpose in most historical investigations, there are often other goals in such projects as well, such as explanation, interpretation and comparison. Similar goals are often pursued in survey, experimental and other quantitatively-oriented studies.

While it is often thought that in historical research, there is no need for establishing hypotheses, whether explicitly stated or implicitly held, to guide and direct the investigation, this is not true of most historical projects in which hypotheses are at the heart of the investigation (Krampitz, 1981, p. 55). Similarly, there is a need to establish reliability and validity within historical designs in order to confirm that the sources from which the data are obtained have provided valid information (Christy, 1975, pp. 190-191). This may be done by employing a variety of techniques, and lends credibility to the work by confirming that the evidence from which the conclusions are drawn is complete and correct. As Christy has stated: 'A historian does not merely use books or articles with old dates, or gleefully use sections of Grandmother's diary, without first testing out the truthfulness of the material' (p. 190). External criticism is necessary to establish the validity of the documents used in the investigation and internal criticism is essential for determining the reliability of information internal to the documents being used.

The approach used in historical designs is, however, considerably more flexible than that used in experimental designs which must provide for rigid control of the experimental conditions. Because the data cannot be generated by the researcher in historical approaches, there is no need to adopt the rigid and inflexible parameters which are necessary under experimental conditions. In fact, a great deal of flexibility may be required simply to locate as well as evaluate important information for the historical project.

Difficulties which are encountered in employing historical methods relate in large measure to locating or gaining access to primary sources of information. It does, however, depend to a considerable extent on the time period under study.

Generally speaking, the more distant the period of time, the more difficult it is to locate primary sources of data. The latter form the primary focus of the historical researcher's quest for information, and are often elusive. When primary sources cannot be found it may be difficult for the investigator to study the topic adequately since important portions of the data may be missing. Christy has aptly stated in this regard, 'The historiographer's weakest position is when he can establish only *possibility*' (1975, p. 192).

Perhaps the most difficult and undoubtedly the most challenging methodological issue which the historical researcher must face is that of determining the meaning of the information of the data collected: 'Interpretation of the facts is a creative process of the investigator, and the meaning of the facts is not inherent in the facts alone' (Christy, 1975, p. 191). The objectivity, judgement and creativity of the researcher are vital elements in this process and will weigh heavily in the quality of the eventual synthesis of data culminating in the written report.

USE OF HISTORICAL METHODS IN NURSING: STATE OF THE ART

Although nurse researchers who use historical methods are few in number as yet, there is a gradually growing collection of historical theses, dissertations, books and monographs appearing on library shelves. A noteworthy investigation conducted in Canada by Professor Margaret Street was the biography of Ethel Johns, a remarkable woman who was appointed Director of the University of British Columbia School of Nursing upon its establishment in 1919, the first university degree program in nursing in Canada. Miss Johns later went on to become the first editor of *The Canadian Nurse* and the search for primary sources of information took the author to many places in Canada and the United States where Miss Johns had lived and worked. It led her to archives and other libraries, to relatives, to minutes and records of organisations, to letters and personal documents, and to the published writings of Miss Johns. To illustrate the power of the primary source of information and the light it can shed on the subject being studied, the following are Miss Johns' words as she appealed to physicians to adopt positive attitudes towards the new university degree program in

nursing before a joint session of the British
Columbia Hospitals Association and the Canadian
Public Health Association in Vancouver in June of
1920:

> To those who are in opposition or in doubt, one
> last word, if there are any of such here: Will
> you not listen to the appeal of those upon
> whose shoulders you yourselves lay such heavy
> burdens? You see so many faults, so many
> blunders in our nursing service. So do we;
> they are not hidden from us. You cannot imag-
> ine why things should not run more smoothly,
> but we can; we know it is because of insuffi-
> cient teaching and supervision. You do not
> realise how complex your own profession has
> become. How can we expect you to realise how
> difficult it is for us, with few of your advan-
> tages, to keep up with the advance shown in
> medicine? (Street, 1973, p. 132).

The recording of the history of nursing in
various geographic regions is beginning to be
undertaken on a systematic basis as more and more
nurses become aware of the importance of preserving
and maintaining records and of presenting an integrated analysis of the historic events which have
shaped the face of nursing. The use of the oral
history, a method of generating historical information is being used more and more and can provide a
considerable amount of data that will assist in the
understanding of documents which form primary and
secondary sources of information. Investigators
who use oral history methods usually seek to interview nursing leaders about their experiences in
certain situations or across a period of time. The
results of this approach may provide data which may
not be available from another source or which may
compliment existing data while providing a unique
perspective on the information. In collecting oral
histories there is the unique opportunity to ask
questions and to delve in greater depth into some
of the areas being discussed by the person being
interviewed. That is not to say that the process
of developing oral histories is an easy matter, for
it may be difficult to gain the cooperation of a
particular nursing leader, or that individual may
not be able to participate in such an interview.
Others may wish neither to be identified nor to
have their thoughts recorded on certain issues for
posterity to view and to judge. Yet another difficulty lies in the degree of accuracy with which

particular individuals are able to recall events which have occurred in the past.

In her history of the School of Nursing at McMaster University entitled, *Twenty-Five Years A-Growing*, Henrietta Alderson made extensive use of the method of oral history. In one instance she interviewed the first Director of the School of Nursing following its establishment in 1946, Miss Gladys Sharpe, who spoke of her reasons for leaving McMaster in 1949 to take a new position:

> I had reached the point where I hadn't the background to do more; I had gone as far as I could; I had done the spadework, which I felt was well and truly done; the basic foundations were sound and it seemed wise to find someone to go on from this point (1976, p. 55).

Later on Alderson asked a faculty member to recall the result of her efforts several years earlier to establish new courses emphasising a greater relationship between theory and practice in clinical nursing in the acute agency and in the community. The faculty member responded in the following way:

> Initially I felt resistance, the pattern was different, we were no longer giving service in return for room and board, the hours of clinical ward duty were shortened and we didn't work shifts; we had assumed full responsibility for teaching, the hospital staff was reluctant to give up what had been their prerogative and I don't think they trusted us in the beginning; they questioned the students to be sure they were getting all they should; but the students did well, they were convinced of the value of the basic philosophy that we were teaching with respect to the mother-child relationship; it was an exciting experience and the students were supportive (p. 159).

Another method of generating data in historical research is to ask for written submissions from individuals who have personally experienced or witnessed certain events. This was the case with the history of nursing in Alberta undertaken by the Alberta Association of Registered Nurses on the occasion of its fiftieth anniversary in 1966. Nurses from all over the province were asked: 'To help retrace the progress of nursing education through the history of their own schools' (Cashman, 1966, p. i). Thousands of nurses wrote letters

about their experiences and provided that author
with the kind of material needed to prepare the
history. Cashman commented on the process as
follows:

> Taking localized history is unsatisfying work.
> The results often seem trivial and disappoint-
> ing and hardly worth the bother. The project
> might well have foundered in grass-roots dis-
> couragement at this point but it didn't. The
> hard-sought information came in, and when it
> was added to the material gathered earlier, the
> story began coming into view (p. i).

As a result there was a great variety of information on nursing in Alberta sent to the AARN which
the author sifted through and analysed, developing
the material around certain themes. One submission
by District Nurse Amy Conroy, who was appointed in
1934 to the post at Pendryl, west of Pigeon Lake,
recorded the following:

> The fact that you can be of service is well
> worth any effort. Sometimes I think of the
> days when I drove a Ford car in the rural
> district examining schools. In the distance I
> could see steep hills and deep coulees and I
> would wonder how I would ever get over them,
> but by feeding a little more gas and holding
> the wheel a bit firmer I was over them almost
> before I knew it. So it will be with any of
> our problems if we just keep going forward (p.
> 205).

In her monograph entitled *A Divine Discontent-
Edith Kathleen Russell: Reforming Educator*, Carpenter worked from the advantage of having been a
student and later a faculty member working under
the guidance of Miss E.K. Russell, the first Director of the Faculty of Nursing at the University of
Toronto (1982). However the advantage might well
have been a disadvantage, had Carpenter not approached the task with openness, objectivity and
the desire to present her subject complete with
strengths and weaknesses. In doing so the portrait
of this remarkable woman comes alive and her words
and actions become meaningful. One can almost feel
the strength and determination of her character in
the words of the note which was found in her desk
following her retirement: 'If I were to be your
leader for the next 10 years I would never be
content with things as they are and I want a

successor more discontented still than I' (Carpenter, 1982, p. iv). Citing her service on a Committee of the International Council of Nurses to study
the facilities in London, England for advanced
nursing education at the mid-point of her career,
Carpenter refers to her submission of a minority
report on the matter as a result of her concern
over generality of the Committee Report:

> The Florence Nightingale International Founda-
> tion shall not rest content with the 'Facili-
> ties in London for advanced nursing education'
> until these facilities include access to at
> least one school of nursing that is independent
> financially, and that is conducting a carefully
> controlled experiment in the general training
> of nurses. This school should give considera-
> tion equally to the work of the hospital nurse
> and the work of the Public Health nurse in
> planning the preparation needed in both fields.
> It is hoped that the special school of nursing
> for which this Report asks will organise itself
> in such a manner that it will be able to under-
> take this research work (1982, pp. 47-48).

Considering that the year in which the above took
place was 1936, Miss Russell's submission of a
minority report would seem to reflect a single-mind-
ed determination to express her views on matters of
importance that must have been uncharacteristic of
the times.

Monteiro (1972) was puzzled by the identity of
a woman who corresponded frequently with Florence
Nightingale, a Miss Marsh. She began to search for
references to this woman whose Christian name was
not used in the correspondence in standard references, in works on Florence Nightingale, and by
following up on information given in the letters
themselves. A reference to a 'Catherine' Marsh was
found in a rather obscure 1887 book on Miss Nightingale and two other women, and this first clue led
to success in obtaining a great deal more information about Catherine Marsh including notices about
her health and finally her death in the London
Times (1972, pp. 526-527). Later Monteiro published a collection of Florence Nightingale's
letters which included those written to Catherine
Marsh, one of which was a reproduction of the
original in Miss Nightingale's handwriting
(Monteiro, 1974). As Christy has observed: 'A
writer of history must develop the curiosity,

perseverance, tenacity, and skepticism of the detective' (1975, p. 192).

Allemang (1974) chose a much broader subject for her historical investigation entitled: *Nursing Education in the United States and Canada - 1873-1950: Leading Figures, Forces, Views on Education.* In reading her work it is apparent that she has approached this study from a broad social perspective, and that this was vital to the understanding of the ideas and themes discussed:

> an economic depression and two world wars brought greater visibility to unmet human needs in rural and urban societies. . . . It is well to note the continuing power of the idea that nursing schools should meet the qualitative and quantitative needs of society. . . . Although these schools were successful in meeting society's immediate need for numbers of nurses, ultimately the results were detrimental to the need for nursing leadership and quality in nursing practice. Thus the next generation of nurses concluded that quality not numbers, must be the primary goal of nursing education (1974, pp. 251-252).

Although a work such as this is a monumental undertaking, it is nevertheless essential that researchers continue to address some of the recurring and important questions which have faced the profession over its history.

In concluding this discussion of the state of the art of historical research in nursing, it can be said that there have been some valuable contributions to the literature by historical researchers in recent years. Also it would appear that interest in this area is increasing as new investigators qualified to undertake such work devote their efforts to historical questions of interest. However continuing 'consciousness raising' and increased emphasis is in order so that value is placed upon the historical in all areas of nursing and in order to heighten the interest of younger professionals to seek advanced preparation in this area. Notter has concluded that:

> A major contribution of historical inquiry is in the development of a broader, more complete perspective to enhance our understanding of the present and our approach to the future. Without this knowledge and perspective we are

continually doomed to rediscovery of the wheel (1972, p. 483).

REFERENCES

Alderson, H.J. (1976). *Twenty-five years a-growing.* Hamilton: McMaster University.

Allemang, M.M. (1974). *Nursing education in the United States and Canada - 1873-1950: Leading figures, forces, views on education.* PhD dissertation, University of Washington.

Ashley J.A. (1978). Foundations for scholarship: Historical research in nursing. *Advances in Nursing Science, 1(1),* 25-36.

Carpenter, H.M. (1982). *A divine discontent - Edith Kathleen Russell: Reforming educator.* Faculty of Nursing, University of Toronto.

Cashman, T. (1966). Heritage of service: The history of nursing in Alberta. The Alberta Association of Registered Nurses.

Christy, T.E. (1975). The methodology of historical research: A brief introduction. *Nursing Research, 24(3),* 189-192.

Hayes, C.J., & Moon, P.T. (1929). *Ancient and medieval history.* New York: The MacMillan Co.

Krampitz, S.D., & Pavlovich, N. (1981). Research design: Historical. In S.D. Krampitz (Ed.), *Readings for nursing research* (pp. 54-58). St. Louis: The C.V. Mosby Co.

Mead, M. (1955). *Male and female.* New York: The New American Library.

Monteiro, L. (1974). *Letters of Florence Nightingale.* Boston: Mugar Memorial Library Nursing Archive.

Monteiro, L. (1972). Research into things past: Tracking down one of Miss Nightingale's correspondents. *Nursing Research, 21(6),* 526-529.

Notter, L.E. (1972). The case for historical research in nursing. *Nursing Research, 21(6),* 483.

Shaver, J.F. (1978). Research and the discipline of
nursing. In C.M. Stainton, J.C. Kerr, & J.
Moore, *Perspectives: Nursing education, prac-
tice and research*. Proceedings of the 1978
Annual Meeting of the Western Region, Canadian
Association of University Schools of Nursing.
Calgary: University of Calgary.

Street, M. (1973). *Watchfires on the mountains: The
life and writings of Ethel Johns*. Toronto:
University of Toronto Press.

Symons, T.H.B. (1975). *To know ourselves: The
report of the Commission on Canadian Studies*.
Ottawa: Association of Universities · and Colleges of Canada.

Chapter Three

NURSING RESEARCH INSTRUMENTS: SOME CONSIDERATIONS AND RECOMMENDATIONS

Mary Jane Ward

Nursing research has come a long way. Even a cursory review of old and new issues of nursing research periodicals, the number and quality of nursing research related texts, the number and types of calls for research papers and the nature of nursing research conference programs provide convincing evidence of the exponential growth in nursing research. As the quantity of nursing research has grown, so too the quality of that research has improved. With more and more nurses acquiring research skills and sharing those skills with others, the patient, the profession and the health care system stand to benefit.

Much of nursing research is at the descriptive and exploratory level. There is a need for this type of research for it provides the basis for sound experimentation. However, in order to establish the scientific basis of nursing and advance the profession, predictive and explanatory studies which include control are needed. Such experimental designs are not easy in the case of nursing research, for the investigator is dealing with human beings and control of many of the variables that exist in nursing situations is not possible. Even in the case of carefully designed studies of nursing intervention outcomes, variables are often difficult to identify and control.

There are, however, examples of successful studies in the literature. Many of them were brought together in the Conduct and Utilization of Research in Nursing Project carried out under the auspices of the Michigan Nurses Association (CURN Project, 1981). Based upon specific criteria and a detailed review of nursing literature, research findings that were ready to be used in nursing practice were identified. The research-generated

knowledge was transformed into protocols which
identified research based principles to guide
practice innovations, directions for implementing
innovations and procedures for evaluating their
effects, i.e., outcomes. Ten research-based protocols were developed and field tested. The protocols included: structured preoperative teaching;
reducing diarrhoea in tube-fed patients; preoperative sensory preparation to promote recovery;
preventing decubitus ulcers; intravenous cannula
change; closed urinary drainage systems; deliberative nursing actions to reduce pain; mutual goal
setting in patient care; clean intermittent catheterization; and using research to improve nursing
practice (CURN Project, 1981).

In designing nursing research projects, the
investigator faces the problem of choosing the best
data collection instrument(s) possible in terms of
the study's population and setting. Before selecting an instrument, the researcher needs background
knowledge about tests and measurement, suggestions
about locating and evaluating already developed
instruments and an overview of the process of
developing an original one. In this chapter, those
concerns are addressed, as is the process of developing a compendium of nursing research instruments,
an undertaking pioneered by the Western Interstate
Commission for Higher Education in Nursing.

INSTRUMENTATION

Instrumentation refers to the process of selecting
or developing tools to collect data for the purpose
of measuring the variables under investigation.
Prior to selecting or developing a research instrument, the researcher ought to understand basic
concepts and principles of measurement. There are
many good references that provide such information,
among them, Glass and Stanley (1970); Hopkins and
Glass (1978); Hopkins and Stanley (1980); Kerlinger
(1973); Polit and Hungler (1983); Waltz and Bausell
(1981); and Williamson (1981).

Armed with knowledge about measurement, the
researcher should become acquainted with and explore the various approaches that can be used to
collect data. These include anecdotal notes;
content analysis; critical incident technique;
decision-making exercises; delphi technique; interviews, both structured and unstructured; tests of
knowledge; audits; observation; paper-and-pencil
approaches such as questionnaires, checklists,

rating scales, and semantic differentials; Q-sort; analysis of existing records such as nursing care plans, incident reports, and nurses' notes; process recording; multimedia techniques; and recording of physiological data. Each of these has its own characteristics, strengths and weaknesses, and other aspects to consider before making a decision as to the one most appropriate for a particular study.

PROPERTIES OF A RESEARCH INSTRUMENT

Whether aimed at answers to specific questions or testing hypotheses, data collection instruments must be valid, reliable and feasible. Whether a new instrument is designed or an existing one is used, it must provide valid and reliable data and be practicable for the study's purposes, population, and setting.

The concepts of validity and reliability, often glibly discussed in relation to data collection instruments, are among the least well understood by many researchers. No instrument is valid and reliable per se. A researcher must establish an instrument's validity and reliability for her/his own study. The fact than an instrument has shown validity and reliability under similar circumstances does add to its credibility, but does not establish those characteristics for all subsequent studies for which it might be used. The question must always be asked: Valid and reliable for what purposes, for what population, for what setting, and under what circumstances?

The concepts of validity and reliability are multifaceted and not unrelated. Validity is the real aim of data collection; reliability is a necessary prerequisite for but does not guarantee validity. However, validity does guarantee some degree of reliability. Stated another way, one can have reliability without validity but one cannot have validity without some degree of reliability. An instrument that cannot be depended upon to give the same results when used (reliability) cannot measure accurately and, therefore, cannot have validity (Suchman, 1970).

The feasibility or practicality of an instrument refers to its usability, and instruments vary widely in this respect. An instrument's feasibility is affected by its economy, that is, its initial costs, any special training required to use it, equipment or supplies entailed, and the time

required for administering, scoring, coding, analysing, and interpreting the data collected. The
importance of this attribute must not be minimized
for the feasibility of the research instrument
plays a vital part in the success or failure of any
project.

EXISTING INSTRUMENTS

One of the primary problems confronted by nurse
researchers relative to a research study is that of
locating appropriate existing instruments or,
failing that, creating instruments to measure the
variables of interest. Beginning steps have been
taken in an effort to alleviate the first problem,
culminating in the publication of *Instruments for
Measuring Nursing Practice and Other Health Care
Variables*, Vol. 1 and 2 (Ward & Lindemann, 1979)
and *Instruments for Use in Nursing Education Research* (Ward & Fetler, 1979). These volumes were
published in an effort to help nurse researchers
locate potential instruments and provide background
information that would assist in judging an instrument's appropriateness for a particular study.

There are other published compilations that
provide useful information on existing instruments
relevant to nursing research. These include:
American Alliance for Health, Physical Education
and Recreation (undated); Beatty (1969); Beere
(1979); Bolton (1976); Bonjean, Hill and McLemore
(1967); Boyer, Simon and Karofin (1973); Buros
(1970, 1974, 1978); Cattell and Warburton (1967);
Chun, Cobb and French (1975); Compton (1980);
Comrey, Backer and Glaser (1973); Cook et al.
(1981); Educational Testing Service (1968); George
and Maddox (1978); Goldman and Saunders (1974);
Goldman and Busch (1979); Goodwin and Driscoll
(1980); Hyman et al. (1978); Johnson and Bomarito
(1971); Johnson (1976); Kane and Kane (1981); Lake,
Miles and Earle (1973); Lyerly (1973); Mardell and
Goldenberg (1972); Miller (1977); Mangen and Petter-
son (1982); Price (1972); Reeder, Ramacher and
Gorelnik (1976); Robinson, Athanasiou and Head
(1969); Robinson, Rusk and Head (1968); Robinson
and Shaver (1973); Shaw and Wright (1967); Simon
and Boyer (1970); Snider and Osgood (1969); Strauss
(1969); Thomas (1970); Walker (1973); and Wylie
(1974).

Many university and specialised research
libraries have files of published tests that have
been subjected to rigourous evaluation; these

constitute an important research resource. It be-
hooves researchers to search systematically the
literature for instruments which may be available
to measure the concepts being studied. Alternate-
ly, revisions or adaptations of existing instruments may be appropriate. Either approach would
add to the knowledge of the psychometric properties
of available instruments and thus would constitute
a scientific contribution.

In examining an existing instrument to determine its appropriateness for a specific research
purpose, certain questions should be addressed.
These include:

1. Regardless of title, exactly *what* does the
    available instrument measure?
2. Are the concepts measured by the instrument
    the same as those the researcher plans to
    investigate?
3. *How* does the instrument measure the concepts
    of interest?
4. What was the theoretical or conceptual basis
    underlying the development of the instrument?
5. What steps were involved in the instrument's
    development? When was it developed? Has it
    been revised? Is it outdated? Is the lan-
    guage current?
6. Are any reliability and validity data avail-
    able? Have norms been established?
7. For what population was the instrument intend-
    ed? On what population(s) was it tested? For
    what population(s) is it appropriate?
8. How is the instrument administered and scored?
    What does the score mean?
9. How long does it take to complete the instru-
    ment? Are directions clear and easily under-
    stood?
10. What resources does the instrument require in
    terms of personnel, skill, time and finances
    to reproduce or purchase, administer, complete
    and score?
11. How has the instrument been used, by whom and
    with what results?
12. What does use of the instrument entail, e.g.,
    obtaining copyright permission, providing a
    copy of original data to the instrument's
    author, sharing publication and/or presenta-
    tion credit, etc.?

Because of high publication costs and the
number of articles awaiting publication, authors
are encouraged to keep their manuscripts brief;

hence, it is often impossible to answer the above questions based on a published article alone. Obtaining this kind of information often requires that one contact the instrument's author, but it is well worth the effort.

Developing a Research Instrument

Creating a research instrument is not a task to be undertaken lightly or without a great deal of thought and planning. The amount of knowledge, work and time required to develop, pretest and refine a worthwhile instrument should not be underestimated. The steps referred to are essential in establishing the instrument's validity, reliability and feasibility. As more nurses become interested in research and aware of the meaning and importance of the concepts of measurement, the quality of research instruments is improving. There are a number of good references available that describe in detail technical aspects of instrument construction (Gay, 1976; Kidder, 1981; Mouly, 1970; Nunnally, 1972; Polit & Hungler, 1983; Wesman, 1971). A brief overview of the process is outlined below for the purpose of emphasising the complexity, resources, work and time involved.

The first steps in the construction of an instrument are those of obtaining a thorough grasp of the field or area under study, the research question, the objectives of the study, the nature of the data sought and how data will be analysed. There is no substitute for careful, detailed planning. Further, the researcher must recognise limits to the demands to be made on subjects in terms of the time and effort needed to answer questions or supply other data for a study. It is important to collect only data essential to answering the research question and to avoid asking for nice to know or interesting to know data.

The choice of a data collection instrument will depend on many factors. However, because of the popularity of the paper-and-pencil questionnaire, a brief overview of the steps in its construction will be used as an example of instrument development. Prepared with in-depth knowledge of the area to be investigated and some knowledge of psychometrics, the researcher should develop a bank of potential items or questions, all of which are eligible for inclusion in the final version of the instrument. The contents of the bank should be based on the researcher's experience, that of peers and acknowledged experts in the area of interest and an extensive literature review. This bank should be reasonably exhaustive and items should be categorised on the basis of the general areas which define or describe the content domain under study.

The categories and the number of items within each category provide guidelines for the number and type of subsections required for the finished instrument, as well as the number of items that should be selected as representative of each category. This step of identifying subsections and the portion of the final instrument which each subsection should represent is often referred to as preparing an instrument blueprint, preparing a table of specifications, model or plan. Such a blueprint or table is fundamental to the process of establishing content validity. Its purpose is to assure that the instrument's items will constitute a representative sample of the total content or domain to be measured.

Once the blueprint is developed, the next step is to choose specific items that are representative of the identified categories; each item selected must be justified on the basis of its contribution to the overall purpose of the research study. Once selected, items should be pretested for clarity, relevance and appropriateness. Nunnally (1978) recommends pretesting with at least five persons per item if at all feasible and conducting the pretest with subjects as representative of the study group as possible.

When the clarity, appropriateness and relevance of each item has been established, the items should be used to create a draft of the total questionnaire. The draft should be pretested with subjects who are similar to those who will constitute the subjects in the proposed study. Pretest results should then be subjected to appropriate statistical procedures to establish the psychometric properties of the instrument. Too often this step is ignored by nurse researchers and others as well. Nurses who do not have the skills needed to undertake this step should seek help by consulting psychometricians, statisticians and/or textbooks on test theory and statistics such as Kerlinger (1973); Winer (1971); Cronbach (1970); Nunnally (1978); Magnusson (1967); Guilford and Fruchter (1973); Hopkins and Stanley (1981); and Thorndike (1971).

The results of the analysis of the psychometric properties of the instrument may lead the researcher to further revisions and/or more

pretesting and analysis or they may indicate that
the instrument is ready for use. How will this be
known? Again, this depends upon the study's purposes, population, setting and circumstances.
Directions must be clear and concise. In developing an instrument it is important insofar as possible to limit measurement to one variable in order
to improve the quality of the instrument. The
emergence of strong and credible instruments to
measure nursing research variables will undoubtedly
facilitate the profession's efforts to develop a
classification system for those instruments (Ward &
Lindeman, 1979, p. 2).

THE NURSING RESEARCH INSTRUMENTS COMPILATIONS PROJECTS

In 1972 the Western Council on Higher Education in
Nursing (WCHEN) of the Western Interstate Commission for Higher Education (WICHE) in Boulder,
Colorado, was awarded a federally-funded Regional
Nursing Research Development Program Grant. One of
the problems identified early in that program was
the difficult, time-consuming task of locating
appropriate research instruments. In 1974 the
Research Branch, Division of Nursing, United States
Department of Health, Education and Welfare
(USDHEW) signed a contract with WICHE as one approach to alleviating the research instrument
problem. The contract stipulated that WCHEN was to
develop and prepare for publication a compilation
of research instruments appropriate for nursing
research. The project began in July 1974 and was
completed in February 1977.

The need for a similar compilation of instruments focusing on nursing education research was
soon apparent. Funds for such a project were
successfully sought from the Special Projects
Grants Section, Division of Nursing, USDHEW. This
project began in March 1977 and was completed in
March 1979, with the posting of 200 copies of a
big, bright red book. Because the process for
completing the projects was much the same, it is so
described with special attention only to major
differences.

Process
Appropriately, staff were charged with the major
responsibility for meeting the objectives by the
two projects. However, Dr. Jo Eleanor Elliott, now

Director, Division of Nursing, United States De-
partment of Health and Human Services (USDHHS); Dr.
Carol Lindeman, Dean, University of Oregon Health
Sciences Center School of Nursing; and Dr. Doris
Bloch, Chief, Research Grants Section, Division of
Nursing, USDHHS, played important roles in the
success of the projects.

Two advisory committees were used during the
first project; one was used during the second. The
three committees included persons from across the
United States, most from nursing, but some from
outside of nursing, who were identified as having
the skills necessary for the projects' success.
Two committees were needed for the first project,
for the resulting compilation included a description of instruments to measure physiological variables and a committee of nurse physiologists was
recruited to guide that effort.

The advisory committees met for two-day sessions twice each year during the life of each
project and telephone conferences were held as
needed. The committees provided guidance and
direction for the projects. They helped staff
develop guidelines, plan project processes, and
make decisions about the actual nature, format and
content of the resulting publications. They helped
set parameters and develop criteria for what was to
be included or excluded from each publication,
reviewed materials, and helped identify strategies
and resource persons whose skills were needed.

First, as Co-Director and later as Director,
this author identified the steps necessary for
completion of the projects, then developed a detailed plan and time chart for each step. Sharing
information about the projects was crucial to their
success. Letters were sent to all deans of schools
of nursing, all deans of graduate schools of nursing and all directors of research offices in
schools of nursing in the United States and Canada.
The letters briefly described the projects and
sought help in identifying persons who had developed or used research instruments that would be
appropriate for the publications. Notices to be
shared with faculty and students and posted on
bulletin boards were included with the letters.

Notices and advertisements about the projects
were placed in appropriate professional journals.
Information about the project was shared at meetings on the local, state, regional, national and
international levels through oral announcements,
posters, and descriptive flyers included in registration packets or placed on registration tables.

Extensive retrospective, current and continuous reviews of literature in nursing and related fields were conducted along with examinations and reviews of compilations in other fields and disciplines. The related fields and disciplines included anthropology, education, medicine, nutrition, physiology, public health, psychology and sociology.

Once an instrument was identified that might be considered for inclusion in the publications, steps were taken to contact the author or nurse researcher who had used it. That person was asked to provide the staff with (1) a copy of the instrument or information as to where a copy could be obtained, (2) a detailed description of the instrument itself following guidelines of a staff-developed form, and (3) a copy of a write-up of the results of a project or study in which the instrument had been used or information about where such material could be obtained.

When these pieces of information had been collected, staff prepared a detailed description of the instrument and its development along with brief annotations of nursing research in which it had been used, copyright information, and the name and address of the person to contact for additional information about using the instrument.

Following a telephone call to notify the contact person (in most cases, the instrument's developer) to be expecting the description and to verify addresses, two copies of the descriptions were sent to these persons for verification of the information contained, any needed updating and suggested changes in the description. If changes were to be substantial, authors were asked to contact staff by telephone. If changes were minor, authors were asked to make them on both copies and return one to staff by mail. If necessary, these steps were repeated until both author and staff were satisfied with the descriptions.

Once this step had been completed, each instrument, each description and all of the information on which the description had been based were reviewed by an experienced nurse researcher and a psychometrician. Appropriate changes suggested by these persons were incorporated into the descriptions by staff and these new drafts were again shared with the authors. Copyright releases and signed *Permission to Publish* forms were obtained from each author or appropriate source, e.g., publisher of a periodical, a book, etc. Staff were responsible for all other portions of the publications that they and the Advisory Committees had agreed would be helpful to users. These included, for example, Table of Contents, Introduction, Indices, Appendices, etc.

For the first project, staff included the Project Director, one full-time secretary and such part-time people as the ebb and flow of the work made necessary. For the second project, the permanent staff included only the Project Director, a staff assistant, and a full-time secretary. A part-time secretary and a contract editor helped with the final preparation of both manuscripts.

The manuscript for the first publication was sent to the Division of Nursing, Washington, D.C., for it was to be printed and distributed by the United States Government Printing Office. (A second printing has been prepared by the Western Interstate Commission for Higher Education to fill the requests for copies.)

Grant stipulations for the compilation of nursing education research instruments provided that WICHE would be responsible for its publication and distribution. Thus, for that volume, staff had additional responsibilities. Camera ready copy and specifications for calls for bids were prepared; bids from publishers were solicited; art work was designed and agreed upon; contracts were signed; blue-line copies were proofed and corrected.

Results

Both reference books became available to the public in March 1979. *Instruments for Measuring Nursing Practice and Other Health Care Variables*, Vol. 1 and 2 contain detailed descriptions, critiques and reproductions of 138 psychosocial research instruments; descriptions of 19 instruments that measure physiological parameters; an annotated bibliography of other selected compilations; a glossary of physiological instrument terms; and a page of suggested electrical safety practices for health care personnel. The publication is indexed by author, instrument title and key terms.

Instruments for Use in Nursing Education Research contains descriptions, critiques and reproductions of 78 instruments; brief descriptions and references for an additional 40 instruments that have been used in nursing education research but were described in other published compilations such as Buros, Comrey, Lake, Miles, etc.; an annotated bibliography of other published instrument

compilations; and a glossary of research and psychometric terms. This publication, too, is indexed
by author, instrument titles, and key terms.

In both books, each description includes key
concepts, title, author, variables measured, nature
and content of the instrument, its administration
and scoring, the rationale for its development, the
source of items, procedures used for the instrument's development, information about reliability
and validity, a brief description of nursing studies in which the instrument has been used, selected
comments about the instrument, references, the name
and address of a person to contact for additional
information and when appropriate, the name of the
copyright owner.*

Suggestions
For anyone or any group considering a similar
undertaking, this author has several suggestions
that will expedite the task:
o   Think through and plan each step of the pro-
     ject carefully and in detail; some alterations
     may have to be made, but hopefully they will
     be minor ones.
o   Identify knowledgeable resource persons early
     and maintain close contact with them.
o   Be open, honest and straight-forward with
     people who submit instruments to be considered
     for the compilation. Our project staff made
     every attempt to do this; it was effective and
     saved a great deal of time. These people
     trusted us not to make changes in the descrip-
     tions and comments about their instruments
     without their being informed. This trust and
     rapport also helped keep names and addresses
     current so that little time was lost when
     there was a need to contact someone.
o   Use the telephone; people seemed to appreciate
     having a voice to associate with the signature
     on a letter. Use of the telephone did much to
     expedite the project work especially when mail
     was involved. A telephone call alerted the
     person to be expecting the material; thus,
     none was ever lost (quite a feat!). Having
     been alerted, the recipient was expecting the
     material and had allowed time to review it.
     Project staff were convinced that this cut
     turn around time considerably.
o   Plan a realistic timetable; remember there may
     be unexpected delays. A paper mill workers'

strike delayed the second of these projects for several weeks.

o   Remember nurses are a very mobile population and change their names through marriage and divorce thus often making the first contact with them time-consuming. Expect to develop some detective-type skills for locating people.

o   Don't underestimate the amount of detail that needs attending to early: forms must be developed; lists of names and addresses accumulated; realistic plans made for the literature review, etc. Careful planning here saves days and weeks later.

o   Plan a realistic budget. It would be devastating to do all of that work only to discover there was no money for publication or making the material available. Explore possible sources of financial assistance for your project. There may well be granting agencies or institutions which would be interested in supporting such an endeavours.

o   Don't lose your sense of humor or perspective! Work on such a project is hard and, at times, frustrating, but it is very educational and it is rewarding personally and professionally. There is a great deal of satisfaction to be gained from having made such a contribution to the nursing profession.

CONCLUSION

This same process could be adapted by nurses in other countries and other regions as a means of sharing and improving research instruments. Each country that has a body of nurse researchers, however small, could establish a library of research instruments. Such libraries could serve as nursing research information clearinghouses. They could contain copies of the instruments themselves and all available information about them: their development; their psychometric properties; their strengths and weaknesses; abstracts of studies, theses, and dissertations in which they have been used, etc. These libraries would be a valuable resource to nurses, students and other researchers of the resident countries and to those of other countries as well. At the moment, even within a single country, it is often very difficult to gain access to such information on research instruments except in the published volumes referred to earlier. The passing of information by word of mouth is simply not good enough today when there is a vast and rapidly developing array of communications technology available to assist with such problems. However, the continuing need to update such materials makes the clearinghouse idea very attractive. In the best of all worlds one would visualize the availability of such information on a computer data bank accessible to researchers all over the world.

Such sharing would make it possible for researchers to devote valuable time to developing and improving psychometrically sound instruments rather than quickly constructing their own which are often of questionable quality.

NOTES

*   These volumes are available from the Western Interstate Commission for Higher Education, Post Office Drawer P, Boulder, Colorado, 80302, U.S.A.

REFERENCES

American Alliance for Health, Physical Education and Recreation (undated). *Testing for impaired, disabled and handicapped individuals.* Washington, DC: Author.

Beatty, W.H. (1969). *Improving educational assessment and an inventory of measures of affective behavior.* Washington, DC: Association for Supervision and Curriculum Development, NEA.

Beere, C. (1979). *Women and women's issues: A handbook of tests and measurements.* San Francisco: Jossey-Bass.

Bolton, B. (Ed.), (1976). *Handbook of measurement and evaluation in rehabilitation.* Baltimore, MD: University Park Press.

Bonjean, C., Hill, R.N., & McLemore, S.D. (1967). *Sociological measurement: An inventory of scales and indices.* San Francisco: Chandler Publishing Company.

Boyer, E.G., Simon, A., & Karofin, G.R. (Eds.), (1973). *Measures of maturation: An anthology of early childhood observation instruments.* Philadelphia: Research for Better Schools.

Buros, O. (Ed.), (1970). *Personality tests and reviews.* Highland Park, NJ: Gryphon Press.

Buros, O. (Ed.), (1978). *Tests in print II.* Highland Park, NJ: Gryphon Press.

Buros, O. (Ed.), (1970). *The eighth mental measurements yearbook.* Highland Park, NJ: Gryphon Press.

Cattell, R., & Warburton, F. (1967). *Objective personality and motivation tests.* Urbana, IL: University of Illinois Press.

Chun, K., Cobb, S., & French, J. (1975). *Measures for psychological assessment: A guide to 3,000 original sources and their application.* Ann Arbor: University of Michigan Institute for Social Research.

Compton, C. (1980). *A guide to 65 tests for special education.* Belmont, CA: Pitman Learning.

Comrey, A., Backer, T., & Glaser, E. (1973). *A sourcebook of mental health measures.* Los Angeles: Human Interaction Research Institute.

Cook, J.D., Hepworth, S.J., Wall, T.D., & Warr, P.B. (1981). *The experience of work. A compendium and review of 249 measures and their use.* New York: Academic Press.

Cronbach, L., & Meehl, P.E. (1955). Construct validity in psychological tests. *Psychological Bulletin, 52,* 281-302.

CURN Project. (1981). *Structured preoperative teaching.* New York: Grune and Stratton.

CURN Project. (1981). *Reducing diarrhea in tube-fed patients.* New York: Grune and Stratton.

CURN Project. (1981). *Preoperative sensory preparation to promote recovery.* New York: Grune and Stratton.

CURN Project. (1981). *Preventing decubitus ulcers.* New York: Grune and Stratton.

CURN Project. (1981). *Intravenous cannula change.* New York: Grune and Stratton.

CURN Project. (1981). *Closed urinary drainage systems.* New York: Grune and Stratton.

CURN Project. (1981). *Pain: Deliberative nursing interventions.* New York: Grune and Stratton.

CURN Project. (1981). *Mutual goal setting in patient care.* New York: Grune and Stratton.

CURN Project. (1981). *Clean intermittent catheterization.* New York: Grune and Stratton.

CURN Project. (1981). *Using research to improve patient care: A guide.* New York: Grune and Stratton.

Educational Testing Services. (1968). *Disadvantaged children and their first school experiences: ETS - head start longitudinal study.* Princeton, NJ: Author.

Gay, L.R. (1976). *Educational research: Competencies for analysis and application.* Columbus, OH: Merrill Publishing Company.

Glass, G., & Stanley, J. (1970). *Statistics in education and psychology* (2nd ed.). Englewood Cliffs, NJ: Prentice-Hall.

Goldman, B.A., & Busch, J.C. (1979). *Directory of unpublished experimental measures* (vol. 2). New York: Human Sciences Press.

Goldman, B.A., & Saunders, J.L. (1974). *Directory of unpublished experimental measures.* New York: Human Sciences Press.

Goodwin, W., & Driscoll, L. (1980). *Handbook for measurement and evaluation in early childhood: Issues, measures and methods.* San Francisco: Jossey-Bass.

Guilford, J.B., & Fruchter, B. (1973). *Fundamental statistics in psychology and education* (5th ed.). New York: McGraw-Hill.

Hopkins, K., & Glass, G. (1978). *Basic statistics for the behavioral sciences.* Englewood Cliffs, NJ: Prentice-Hall.

Hopkins, K., & Stanley, J. (1981). *Educational and psychological measurement and evaluation* (6th ed.). Englewood Cliffs, NJ: Prentice-Hall.

Hyman, R.B., Woog, P., & Farrell, H.K. (1978). *Current non-projective instruments for the mental health field.* New York: Atcom.

Johnson, O. (1976). *Tests and measurements in child development: Handbooks I and II.* San Francisco: Jossey-Bass.

Johnson, O., & Bommarito, J. (1971). *Tests and measurements in child development: A handbook.* San Francisco: Jossey-Bass.

Kane, R.A., & Kane, R.L. (1981). *Assessing the elderly: A practical guide to measurement.* Lexington, MA: Lexington Books.

Kerlinger, F. (1973). *Foundations of behavioral research* (2nd ed.). New York: Holt, Rinehart & Winston.

Kidder, L. (1981). *Selltig, Wrightsman and Cook's research methods in social relations* (4th ed.). New York: Holt, Rinehart & Winston.

Lake, D., Miles, M., & Earle, R. (1973). *Measuring human behavior.* New York: Teachers College Press.

Lyerly, S. (no date). *Handbook of psychiatric rating scales.* Rockville, MD: National Institutes of Mental Health.

Magnusson, D. (1967). *Test theory.* Palo Alto, CA: Addison-Wesley.

Mangen, D.J., & Peterson, W.A. (Eds.), (1982). *Research instruments in social gerontology* (vols. 1 & 2). Minneapolis, MI: University of Minnesota Press.

Miller, D. (1977). *Handbook of research design and social measurement* (3rd ed.). New York: David McKay Company.

Mouly, G. (1970). *The science of educational research* (2nd ed.). New York: Litton Educational Publishing.

Nunnally, J.C. (1972). *Educational measurement and evaluation* (2nd ed.). New York: McGraw-Hill.

Nunnally, J.C. (1978). *Psychometric theory* (2nd ed.). New York: McGraw-Hill.

Polit, D., & Hungler, B. (1983). *Nursing research: Theory and practice* (2nd ed.). Philadelphia: J.B. Lippincott.

Price, J. (1972). *Handbook of organizational measurement*. Lexington, MA: D.C. Heath.

Reeder, L., Ramacher, L., & Gorelnik, S. (1976). *Handbook of scales and indices of health behavior*. Pacific Palisades, CA: Goodyear Publishing Company.

Robinson, J., Athanasiou, R., & Head, K. (1969). *Measures of occupational attitudes and occupational characteristics*. Ann Arbor: University of Michigan Institute for Social Research.

Robinson, J., Rusk, J.G., & Head, K. (1968). *Measures of political attitudes*. Ann Arbor: University of Michigan Institute for Social Research.

Robinson, J., & Shaver, P. (1973). *Measures of social psychological attitudes*. Ann Arbor: University of Michigan Institute for Social Research.

Shaw, M., & Wright, J. (1967). *Scales for the measurement of attitudes*. New York: McGraw-Hill.

Simon, A., & Boyer, E.G. (1970). *Mirrors for behavior: An anthology of observation instruments*. Philadelphia: Research for Better Schools.

Snider, J.G., & Osgood, C.E. (Eds.). (1969). *Semantic differential technique*. Chicago: Aldine Publishing.

Stanley, J. (1971). Reliability. In R.L. Thorndike (Ed.), *Educational measurement* (2nd ed.). Washington, DC: American Council on Education.

Strauss, M. (no date). *Family measurement techniques: Abstracts of published instruments,*

1935-1965. Minneapolis: University of Minnesota Press.

Suchman, E.A. (1967). *Evaluative research, principles and practices in public service and social action programs.* New York: Russell Sage Foundation.

Thomas, H. (1970). Psychological assessment instruments for use with human infants. *Merrill-Palmer Quarterly, 16,* 179-223.

Thorndike, R.L. (Ed.) (1971). *Educational measurement* (2nd ed.). Washington, DC: American Council on Education.

Thorndike, R.L. (1976). Reliability. In B. Bolton (Ed.), *Handbook of measurement and evaluation in rehabilitation.* Baltimore: University Park Press.

Walker, D. (1973). *Socioemotional measures for preschool and kindergarten children.* San Francisco: Jossey-Bass.

Waltz, C., & Bausell, R.B. (1981). *Nursing research: Design, statistics, and computer analysis.* Philadelphia: F.A. Davis.

Ward, M.J., & Fetler, M. (1979). *Instruments for use in nursing education research.* Boulder, CO: WICHE.

Ward, M.J., & Lindeman, C. (1979). *Instruments for measuring nursing practice and other health care variables* (Vol. 1 & 2). Washington, DC: Superintendent of Documents.

Wesman, A.G. (1971). Writing the test item. In R.N. Thorndike (Ed.), *Educational measurement* (2nd ed.). Washington, DC: American Council on Education.

Williamson, Y. (1981). *Research methodology and its application to nursing.* New York: Wiley and Sons.

Winer, B.J. (1971). *Statistical principles in experimental design* (2nd ed.). New York: McGraw-Hill.

Wylie, R. (1974). *The self-concept: A review of methodological considerations and measuring instruments.* Lincoln, NE: University of Nebraska Press.

Chapter Four

TRANSCULTURAL NURSING RESEARCH: PROCESS, PROBLEMS AND PITFALLS

Janice M. Morse

The purpose in this chapter is to explore the process, problems and pitfalls of clinical nursing research in different cultural settings. These settings may be found either within one's own country, or across international boundaries. There are few nurse researchers engaged in clinical research, and still fewer conducting transcultural clinical nursing research. Although this chapter may appear to be a rather specialised chapter, it is written in the hope of stimulating research in this area, and to serve as a guide for nurse researchers preparing to enter a transcultural setting. It will also explain, for the purposes of grant review, why the same criteria cannot be used to evaluate cross-cultural ethnographic research as is used for evaluating more quantitatively-oriented experimental studies.

The transcultural nurse researcher has a major contribution to make towards the improvement of nursing care. Research involving different racial or cultural groups can provide insights into many nursing problems, but the potential contribution of this research to nursing care is only beginning to be recognised. A few examples of areas in which transcultural nursing research can make a substantial contribution are: the examination of the patient's response to pain, to compliance, and to cultural barriers to care.

Because of the embryonic state of cross-cultural investigation into clinical nursing research, there is scant literature available. The information for this chapter was drawn from several sources. The author has drawn from her own research experiences within the United States and in Fiji, and from the experiences of colleagues involved in this type of research. Anthropological literature was also used, although it is recognised that anthropological research occurs in a different context and for a different purpose than transcultural nursing research. The focus of clinical nursing research is narrower, since it deals with health-related problems rather than with entire communities as in the traditional ethnographic research settings. The nurse researcher must attempt to access formalised bureaucracies within highly structured and often authoritarian hospital and/or government environments. Alternatively, the nurse may choose to work outside the hospital system, studying traditional healers whose practice may or may not be condoned by the government. As a consequence, the transcultural nurse researcher often must operate under greater restrictions than the anthropologist.

For convenience, this chapter is divided into sections according to phases in the research *process*, such as selecting a site, identifying a problem, necessary groundwork prior to departure, and so forth. Finally, although this chapter may appear to be a "shopping-list" type of guide, it is by no means intended to be all-inclusive, nor applicable to all situations.

Identification of a Problem and Research Setting

The identification of a research problem within another culture may be extremely difficult. The question often arises "How can a problem be formulated if one does not know what is *there?*" Thus, the selection of a problem and a research setting may or may not be interrelated, depending on a number of factors. As with all research, the research question arises from the researcher's interests, concerns and prior experiences, but the question once chosen may or may not limit the culture or the geographic location of the research. For example, if the question involves a culture-bound syndrome (e.g., *susto* in Hispanic America, or *latch* in South East Asia), then the research involved would be conducted in those regions.

Sometimes the illness or syndrome to be examined is prevalent in many regions, or in many cultures. Problems concerning, for instance, human adaptation to high altitude must be conducted in areas that are above a certain elevation, and examination of longevity must be conducted in regions in which the inhabitants live longer than in other populations. Occasionally special sociocultural environmental characteristics of a region will provide special conditions for research. The cultural dualism of Fiji, for example, with the limited cultural borrowing between the Fijians and the Fiji-Indians, provided a situation in which two cultures share one ecological environment and one health care system. Thus, differences between the two groups can be maximally attributed to cultural and genetic differences, a situation ideal for comparative studies.

In some cases, selection of a research site may depend on a multitude of other factors. Prior knowledge of a setting is a legitimate reason to select a particular site for research, and hopefully a factor that will ease the problem of identifying a meaningful and feasible research question. The guidance of a mentor (who may already be established in an area), while limiting the new researcher's options, may make the entry process much simpler. Agar (1980) observed that many noted anthropologists obtained their first field experiences examining topics which were not their first choice but rather because their mentors were already engaged in fieldwork in those regions.

Lastly, something as simple as the "itchy feet" syndrome--the desire to travel or to explore a particular culture or region--is an adequate rationale for selecting a region to explore. From the extensive reading that frequently accompanies such daydreaming, researchable questions become increasingly easy to identify.

After much soul-searching and having made the decision to pursue a particular question, it is advisable to examine the chosen country or region for factors which may perhaps make research impossible or intolerable in that setting. Is the country politically unstable or volatile? Are the relations poor between the host country and the country of origin? An affirmative response to either of these questions should result in a serious reconsideration regarding the research site. Poor international relations may prevent the researcher from obtaining the necessary visas and research permits to enter the country, may result in an extremely stressful stay in that country, or may force an early withdrawal prior to the completion of the data collection. Any of these outcomes would be disastrous.

Another more subtle problem may occur if, at the community level, the indigenous people view the external researcher as an intruder or an undesirable alien, so that an extraordinary length of time to gain the trust of the informants would be required before meaningful data could be collected. The accessibility of the research subjects should also be considered. Many governments now feel that it is their responsibility to protect both the culture and the people of unacculturated tribes from exposure to outsiders.

Another concern is the language or dialect spoken in the region. It should be considered whether one's fluency in the language is adequate for interviewing purposes, or if not, whether the necessary conversational level can be acquired within the time constraints of the research. A possible alternative is the use of an intermediate language (such as Pidgin English), or the employment of suitable people to aid in translation and interpretation.

Having selected a geographic area, culture and research topic, it is advisable for the researcher to examine the topic from the perspective of the cultural context in which the research is to be conducted. One should consider whether the research topic is culturally discussible. Will the researcher be able to obtain information on the topic, or will local norms prohibit the discussion? An example of information which may be inaccessible or awkward to research is ritualistic secret information, such as herbal cures used to induce abortion. Such material, even if the researcher does gain access, often can not be ethically disclosed without violating confidentiality, perhaps jeopardising the group and one's reputation as a field-worker.

Will the researcher's gender interfere with the collection of data? For example, cultures vary in their perception of the naturalness of childbirth and sexual matters. One culture may openly share details of these behaviours within their cultures with males and children, while others may only give this knowledge to married females. Thus, information on birthing rituals may or may not be shared with the researcher, depending on the researcher's marital status, age, and the cultural attitudes of the group.

In addition, expected sex-role behaviours frequently interfere with data collection, so that female researchers are given data which the culture thinks women *should* know, while male researchers would be prohibited from gaining access to that same knowledge. Many anthropologists have recognised this dilemma (for example, see Golde, 1970). Prior to the 1960's the majority of anthropological fieldworkers were male, so that information on the women in the society being examined was often sketchy and incomplete. The converse was true for women fieldworkers: Bowen (1964, p. 79) noted that early in her fieldwork she was initially associated with and included only in the activities of the women. She realised that if she remained in a woman's role she would leave the field with "copious information on domestic knowledge without any knowledge of anything else."

The segregation of activities within a community according to gender may impede or prohibit research. One researcher intended to study alcoholism in a developing country, but after her arrival she found that excessive drinking was largely a problem confined to males in that society. As most of the drinking took place in bars that denied entry to women, her access to the research setting made the scope of the topic too limited to be feasible. Some fieldworkers overcome this sort of problem by entering the field as a team (often as husband and wife) so that information from both the male and the female world-views may be obtained.

Foreseeable Problems with Research Methods
Recognition of unique characteristics within the population may determine to some extent the feasibility of the proposed methods. If the population is not literate, this factor alone may preclude many types of data collection, such as the use of questionnaires and pencil-and-paper psychological tests.

Health assessment procedures may have to be modified, since the collection of samples may not be possible. Some Third World cultures believe, for example, that the amount of blood in the body is finite, and that withdrawing even a small sample will result in permanent weakening, since this blood will not be replaced. Baker (1976, p. 13) writes that the Quechua population (in the highlands of Peru) were so resistant to the giving of blood samples that it was "unwise to attempt subcutaneous temperature measurements with a needle probe." Furthermore, this aversion transferred to the taking of blood pressure, which was thought to be due to the unfortunate name of the procedure. The natives suspected that the cuff would extract blood when inflated. The resistance to these procedures resulted in severe limitations to Baker's study of gene systems and blood chemistry.

Many cultures may also be reluctant to give blood or bodily excrement for analysis, but for a different reason. The giving of parts of oneself to a stranger leaves one particularly vulnerable, they believe, for the specimen may be used for sorcery or witchcraft which can cause illness or death. Alternatively, other cultural values may interfere with the measurement or physical examination of the subject. For instance, the head is considered a sacred part of the body by many peoples. Merely touching the head would be considered a very rude behaviour, and may not be culturally permissible, a factor seriously restricting physical measurements.

Finally, the other areas which may restrict data collection are related to the feasibility of moving equipment to the research site, to the operation of this equipment in the field, the extent of facilities available in the area, and the complexity of the analysis. With some types of work this is a less serious problem: researchers undertaking large-scale projects involving multiple personnel and extensive equipment (for example, overland vehicles to transport heavy items) are in a better position than those who must backpack all equipment and supplies into the area. If procedure for analysis is simple and requires little equipment, this may not be a problem. Hemoglobin, for example, can be measured with some degree of accuracy with a hand-held hemoglobinometer, or slides may be prepared in the field and stored for later analysis. However, the measurement of hematocrit is more difficult, as centrifuges are heavy, bulky, and require a power source. Some hand-held models are available, but they do not operate fast enough to separate the plasma nor will they hold a capillary tube. Often refrigeration for the preservation of specimens is not possible, and adverse climates may be the final insult to electric equipment that has been trekked over rough roads. As breakdowns are common, and reagents may spoil, backup contingency plans are essential. In developing countries even the most basic supplies are often either unavailable or else incredibly expensive. An affiliation with a hospital or a clinic in a developing country does not necessarily resolve these problems. The hospital may not always have the equipment, supplies, or the personnel to assist with analysis. It is possible that the barest essentials do not exist, or the hospital cannot permit the use of such scarce resources for frivolous research use by outsiders. These constraints limit and frequently determine the type of data collected.

Groundwork

The first task in understanding the group into which one is to enter is to become acquainted with the culture through the literature, that is, by reading extensively into the history, geography and culture of the host country. It is important, however, to read critically as some of the literature will be of immense value, while other literature will be of no use at all, being biased, irrelevant, outdated, erroneous or contradictory.

Given the mobility of today's world, it is possible that living within the researcher's immediate home-community will· be migrants from the region to which travel is planned. One should seek out such people, requesting assistance as informants and language tutors. These people may also be able to provide contacts in their country.

The importance of establishing contacts, perhaps a fellow researcher or sponsoring agency in the host country, cannot be underestimated. Frequently a government will not provide the researcher with a visa or a research permit unless such support has been obtained (Agar, 1980). If one is unsure how to make this contact, then general letters of inquiry may be written to university social science departments and to the nursing and medical associations in the proposed area. These letters need only make a general statement of the research purpose and plan; proposals need not be included, but may be sent at a later date.

At this stage, contact with other ethnographers who have worked in the same region is an excellent idea. Write or telephone, requesting their feedback on the feasibility of the proposed research, and, if possible, obtain letters of introduction from them. International organisations, such as the World Health Organization, can provide excellent and influential contacts especially if they are active in the region. It is essential that one should collect letters of introduction from important people. Students should seek letters not only from a research adviser, but also from the dean and the university president, as well as from any provincial and local politicians. As these letters are often retained by those to whom they are first presented, it is wise to take additional copies. The importance of such letters for gaining co-operation cannot be overemphasised.

One must not neglect to inquire into the health requirements for a visa, obtain the necessary immunizations, and apply for a passport. Freilich (1970) presents an excellent summary of this process. He notes that obtaining permission from the government to conduct research may be a lengthy and difficult procedure, so that preliminary requests should begin as early as possible. During the past decade governments have become increasingly wary of the involvement of and/or investigations by anthropologists in their countries as a result of several serious breaches of professional ethics. Yet, to approach the government as a *nurse* may result in the government's ignoring, or immediately refusing, the request. To date, in many countries, for a nurse to request permission to do *research* is to request permission to perform a function outside the normal role of the nurse, and from the governmental perspective perhaps incomprehensible.

Decision-making within the government involved may not be the same as that used in the western world. In western countries, the process may be something like this: requests are submitted to the appropriate department, and a committee meets to consider the application according to its merit. Decisions are made to support or to reject the application. In other cultures decision-making may follow other models. Decisions may be made according to the whims or interests of an autocrat, according to the influence of the applicant's relatives and friends, or perhaps, from perceived obligations owed by the host country to the applicant's own country, and so forth. Furthermore the procedure for obtaining permission under such circumstances is also different. Johanson and Edey (1981, p. 150) write that obtaining permission for the removal for the *Lucy* fossils from Ethiopia took one week of visiting offices of dignitaries in the Government of Ethiopia, and drinking endless cups of coffee. The important point is that permission could not be obtained prior to their arrival in Ethiopia. Review boards and funding agencies may find such risks extremely disconcerting, and consider them sufficient reason for refusing funding. But research in a different cultural setting must be conducted using different rules. The risks are higher, but often the results are unique, surprising, and could not otherwise be obtained from working within one's own culture.

Because of the geographical remoteness of many field sites, the researcher, especially the student

researcher, may feel suddenly isolated in the
field, separated from the usual supports of a
library, the consultation of an advisory committee,
and the psychological support of colleagues. Some
floundering from indecision may occur, especially
if the research methods have to be changed. However,
er, if the research question has to be reformulated,
ed, and if the research site is remote enough to
exclude telephone calls for advice, the experience
can be most disconcerting.

Some of these uncertainties can be prevented.
At the literature review stage, photocopy all
pertinent material and summarise books so that
information and references may be taken into the
field, along with a computer-based annotated bibliography. Then, if the question has to be reformulated, the researcher may still be fairly confident
that research will not be duplicating another
study. A support person at home constantly monitoring the literature is also an asset, reducing
the researcher's isolation and fear of reinventing
the wheel.

Proposal Preparation
The preparation of the proposal is usually the most
difficult part of the project, and yet the most
crucial for funding. The researcher becomes involved in a Catch-22 situation, asking: How can I
write a proposal with all the variables clearly
delineated, when I don't know what is *there* before
I arrive? Funding agencies demand a tight proposal, and frequently deny monies for ethnographic,
inductive research on the basis of vagueness. Agar
(1980, pp. 175-183) points out that, at least for
the moment, the experimental design-oriented reviewers hold the purse strings. These persons
(perhaps typically from the field of medicine if
reviewing a health-related nursing proposal) must
therefore be convinced that the inductive, ethnographic approach is worthy of funding. A brief
description of the methodology, using the three
standard buzz-words, participant observation,
ethnographic interview, and field notes, is totally
inadequate. Agar (1980), speaking from his extensive experience as a grant reviewer, recommends
that the process of data collection be discussed in
detail, including an explanation into the inappro-
priateness of the hypothesis-testing approach in
the proposed setting. It is the responsibility of
the proposer to convince the granting agency that

ethnography is not a default option, and that fieldwork is more than a rather pleasant holiday.

Informed consent is rather a sticky problem that must be confronted at this stage. The author's own experience revealed the absurdity of attempting to utilise a consent form which contained all the required components of American informed consent in a Third World setting. In this case, the consent form was complete with statements concerning voluntary participation, withdrawal and so forth. Written in English and translated into two other languages, it filled two legal-sized pages and took a week to prepare in the field. Also this form was for use in a culture that was partly illiterate, and one in which most women themselves did not give consent for their own hospital treatments. Rather, in this patrilineal culture, a form containing one sentence: "I hereby consent to any treatment that the doctor considers necessary" was signed by the patient's husband or father. Fortunately, in January 1981 this requirement for international research was reviewed, so although this issue is still being debated, this form may no longer be necessary (New Regulations on Human Subjects, 1981).

One final word before leaving home: pack some home comforts, and something to withdraw into, such as some favorite books, to help ease the tension when culture shock becomes overwhelming. Even experienced fieldworkers, such as Elenore Bowen (1964) and Margaret Mead (Romanuci-Ross 1980, p. 308) have felt the need for this kind of retreat.

Entering the Research Setting
The period of contact on arrival is frequently filled with unforeseen problems that are added burdens to an already stressful period. It is wise, therefore, to allow plenty of time (much more than would normally be anticipated) and to be patient. One must work closely with administrators, and walk the delicate tightrope of being both visible, low-keyed and non-threatening. Being identified as a nurse will often immediately give the researcher access to information that would usually be inaccessible to the anthropologist. For example, informants will offer personal health information more readily than to a non-medical researcher. One disadvantage, however, is that other information required that is perceived by the informants to be irrelevant or unimportant will not be as easily obtainable. Informants initially

decide what to reveal on what *they* think the researcher wants to know.

Conflict between the researcher's agenda and the government's, or hospital's perception of what a nurse should be or should do may also be awkward. For example, on one occasion the author was not encouraged to apply for a nursing license, for the government perceived the task of research to be outside the domain of nursing.

In doing research, yet another ethical conflict arises for the nurse. It is practically impossible to do hands on nursing *and* at the same time to observe, interview and write field notes. Nursing, especially in countries of limited resources, makes demands on the nurse's attention, focusing the nurse on the tasks at hand, rather than on the larger milieu. Yet, on the other hand, how can a nurse morally and ethically stand by and watch when there is so much to be done and circumstances are clearly desperate?

The last problem to be discussed in this section concerns entering the research setting as a participant observer, and learning the ropes--a stage that has been dubbed rope burns by Sanders (1980). There are numerous stories that circulate at every anthropological meeting about fieldworkers unable to cope with the stress of developing a niche and who spend their time in the field hiding in a hotel reading novels. Entry is a stressful process, rather like leaving a high diving board. However, with few exceptions it gets easier as time progresses, and it is a stage that all fieldworkers must experience (see, for example, Henry & Saberwal, 1969; Kimball & Watson, 1972).

Collection of Data: Problems in the Clinical Areas
While conducting research in the social setting one encounters problems not found in traditional laboratory-based research. In the first place, the researcher has little control over the social settings. The researcher is essentially a guest in this setting (welcomed or tolerated by the participants) rather than the creator or director of research as in the laboratory arena. Furthermore, with ethnographic research the aim of the research is to document the total context. The confusion, the lack of control, the multiple variables are all a part of the naturalistic setting as the purpose is to conduct the research with minimal disruption. There is also a much greater likelihood that unforeseen modifications in the initial proposal

might be required. Because the researcher has little control over the social setting, such problems may even require alteration of the research question itself. Modification of research design may be required due to the lack of subject participation or co-operation, or to problems associated with equipment failure.

These changes, it appears, happen to everyone. One should document the problems that justify the changes and proceed. It is important to maintain regular communication with advisory committees and with funding agencies at home. They should be kept aware of the problems with which the researcher is coping.

When the setting is culturally different from the researcher's own, the process of conducting research becomes even more complex. Language barriers and differing cultural norms make the settings more difficult to analyse, and it is therefore harder to recognise problem areas and to identify solutions. The researcher must therefore acquire the unique ability to remain focused on the research question yet, be adaptable enough to change the methods or to utilise multiple methodologies to seek answers to the research question. If secondary examination of the setting shows the question to be inappropriate or the methods not feasible, one must be able to rephrase or reformulate the question so that it is possible to attain the research goals.

The use of interpreters may be essential for communication, and this introduces the tricky problem of culturally appropriate reimbursement. It is likely that offers of monetary reimbursement will be rigorously refused, leaving the researcher in an awkward reciprocal position (from the researcher's cultural position, at least). Gifts may be substituted, or the salary funds donated to a hospital in a block sum. Carefully examine the culture for clues as to what seems to be appropriate.

As a guest in a hospital, often an uninvited guest at that, finding a space in which to work may initially seem impossible. Wards may be crowded and the beds close together, providing little privacy for interviewing, and even finding a place to write notes may be difficult. Time may be a problem as well as space: a rigid ward schedule may clash with the researcher's schedule. These problems must be dealt with and somehow overcome, but as they are all situation-specific, there are no general solutions to recommend. A combination of tact and perseverance is about all that can be suggested.

The most precious product of the field work experience is data, including the pages of field notes and the tape recordings. In the field it is possible that they may be lost or destroyed: hurricanes occur, roofs leak, and rats and insects destroy papers. It is even possible for the notes to be seized when the researcher is leaving the country, or lost in missing luggage during air travel. The uncertain nature of these conditions show that it is *vital* to make copies of all notes, and to mail immediately (and frequently) these copies to a resource person in the home country. Tape-recorded interviews should be transcribed as soon as possible following the interview for the purpose of analysing data and clarifying any crucial points while it is still possible to reinterview subjects.

Sources of invalidity occur in transcultural research just as in other research, and may, in fact, be increased. The Hawthorne effect--or the change in the subjects behaviour which may be attributed to being observed by the researcher--may be greatly enhanced. In a different culture, especially where the people are less *blase* about research, it is exceedingly difficult for the researcher to blend into the setting. Further, as with all research, the accuracy of official records cannot be assumed. For example, in illiterate populations patients frequently do not know their age, so that an approximate age may be entered into the records which is not indicated as such.

The patient's reporting of symptoms may also prove unreliable, with varying cultural norms interfering with the expected response. For example, when the researcher inquires about the patient's perception of fatigue in a population in which anaemia is endemic, such fatigue may be simply denied. It is possible that these people have always been anaemic, have always been tired, and may not, therefore, recognise lassitude as abnormal.

Conclusion

This chapter constitutes an attempt to illustrate the process, problems, and pitfalls that are peculiar to, or are increased when field work is conducted in transcultural settings. Because the researcher cannot anticipate problems and has little control, compromises frequently have to be made in the research design, in the collection of data, and in the scope of the research. However, in spite of all these difficulties, this type of research may reveal unique insights into problems which would be impossible in the researcher's own culture; thus the value of such studies must not be underestimated. Research in these settings is not easy, and requires stamina, creativity and flexibility. As Rosalie Wax (1971) stated:

> The person who cannot abide feeling awkward or out of place, who feels crushed whenever he makes a mistake-- embarrassing or otherwise-- who is psychologically unable to endure being, and being treated like a fool...ought to think twice before he decides to become a participant observer.

REFERENCES

Agar, M.H. (1980). *The Professional Stranger: An Informal Introduction to Ethnography.* New York: Academic Press.

Baker, P., & Little, M.A. (1976). (Eds.) *Man in the Andes: A Multidisciplinary Study of the High Altitude Quechua.* Strousburg, Penn.: Bowden Hutchinson.

Bowen, E.S. (1964). *Return to Laughter.* New York: Doubleday & Co. Ltd.

Cohen, C., Langness, L.L., Middleton, J., Uchendu, V.C., & Vanstone, J.W. (1970). Entree into the field. In: *A Handbook of Method in Cultural Anthropology.* R. Naroll & R. Cohen (Eds.) New York: Columbia University Press.

Freilich, M. (1970). (Ed.), *Marginal Natives: Anthropologists at work.* New York: Harper & Row, Publ.

Golde, P. (1970). (Ed.), *Women in the Field.* Chicago: Aldine Publ. Co.

Henry, F. & Saberwal, S. (1969). (Eds.) *Stress and Response in Fieldwork.* New York: Holt, Rinehart and Winston.

Johanson, D.C. & Edey, M.A. (1981). *Lucy: The Beginnings of Humankind.* New York: Simon and Schuster.

Kimball, S.T., & Watson, J.B. (1972). (Eds.) *Crossing Cultural Boundaries: The Anthropological Experience.* San Francisco: Chandler Publishing Co.

New Regulations on Human Subjects. (1981). *Anthropology Newsletter, 22:* 8.

Romanucci-Ross, L. (1980). Anthropological Field Research: Margaret Mead, Muse of the clinical experience. *American Anthropologist, 82:* 304-317.

Sanders, C.R. (1980). Ropeburns: Impediments to the achievement of basic comfort early in the field research experience. In: *Fieldwork Experience: Qualitative Approaches to Social Research.* Shaffir, W.B., Stebbins, R.A. & Turowetz, A. (Eds.) New York: St. Martins Press, pp. 158-171.

Wax, R. (1971). *Doing Fieldwork: Warnings and Advice.* Chicago: University of Chicago Press.

PART II: SCIENCE POLICY, HEALTH RESEARCH AND NURSING RESEARCH FUNDING

Chapter Five

HEALTH SCIENCE POLICY AND HEALTH RESEARCH FUNDING IN CANADA

Valerie Wilmot

In this chapter, attention is first drawn to science policy and health research. The focus then shifts to the new federal expenditure management system, the rationale being that it is within these central contexts that any change in the level or type of federal support for nursing research would have to take place.

SCIENCE POLICY[1]

The Evolution of Federal Science Policy

For the past 60 or more years the federal government has played a leading role in encouraging the application of scientific activities to the pursuit of national goals. The potential value of science to society was clearly recognised in the establishment, in 1916, of a Committee of the Privy Council on Scientific and Industrial Research and, at the same time, an Honorary Advisory Council for Scientific and Industrial Research. The Advisory Council, which has since been renamed the National Research Council, was broadly representative of both government and private scientific interests. In the words of one of the Council's later presidents, the Council soon discovered that there was little scientific or industrial research in Canada on which to advise; it therefore set about to establish its own laboratories and to institute programs of support to build up both industrial and university research capability and increase the supply of research scientists trained in the natural sciences in Canada. Meanwhile, other federal departments and agencies were also founding and expanding their own research facilities and, in a limited way, inaugurated a variety of programs for supporting or procuring university research and for ensuring a supply of research-trained scientists in fields related to their own missions.

As early as 1938 the National Research Council had begun to institute special programs of support for medical research and, by 1960, had created a sub-entity called the Medical Research Council. This became a separate body in 1969. With the creation, in 1957, of the Canada Council, to promote and support the arts, humanities and social sciences, the federal structure needed to provide the infrastructure of a national research capability in all disciplines was completed.

As mentioned above, underlying the initial creation of the National Research Council was the notion that it would help the government to foster the rational use of science and technology in pursuit of national goals. This general statement can be said to be the essence of science policy.

Science policy itself, however, has been a matter of vigourous debate in the decade following the mid 60's. The roots of the debate can be traced to the conflict that often arises between those who recognise the evident and tremendous power that science can bring to the solution of real and pressing problems and those who believe that significant advances in knowledge do not occur on command in response to societal needs but happen, sometimes fortuitously, in the context of diligent and painstaking search. The former point to the success of concerted ventures such as the development of the atomic bomb; the latter to such curiosity-motivated discoveries as those of penicillin and insulin or to the theories of Sigmund Freud. To some extent, the conflict lies between those who believe that most of the knowledge already exists to solve some of our important problems and that a concerted effort to fill in the remaining gaps will help to achieve significant ends, and all those who feel that, no matter how much we know now, there is always more to be discovered and the ultimate benefits of what may, at present, seem to be tilting at windmills cannot be fully comprehended but will probably be immense.

Against this background of debate, the government of Canada undertook one of the most extensive reviews of science policy (here defined as the totality of overt decisions specifically involving scientific activities) ever mounted anywhere in the world.

The Senate of Canada, over 15 years ago, set up a Special Committee to receive testimony and briefs from scientists and users of science in every corner of Canada and eventually wrote a four-volume report.[2] It concluded that over the preceding 60 years Canadian science had become too concentrated in government laboratories and universities and too removed from the real problems facing Canada and was, consequently, not fulfilling its potential role in achieving national goals. It therefore made many recommendations aimed at correcting this situation. The fourth volume was published a few years later and described the then status of its recommendations.

The government, meanwhile, established, first, a Science Secretariat within the Privy Council Office, and shortly afterward the Science Council of Canada; in 1971, it transformed the Science Secretariat into the Ministry of State for Science and Technology (MOSST). Both bodies were, at first, advisory in function: the Science Council was composed of acknowledged leaders in science, both academic and industrial, and had a staff of scientific experts; the MOSST was staffed by many public service scientists and science managers, though many scientists were also recruited from outside the public service. The roles of both agencies have been differentiating over the years.

The Science Council is charged with informing the Canadian public about science and related matters and the Ministry is charged with advising the government on matters involving science policy and assisting in the co-ordination of the federal government's own scientific activities, conducted or supported by its many departments and agencies. For a time, the ambit of its advice gradually extended from concern with only the natural sciences and engineering to include exploratory concern with the social sciences. With the advent of the Policy and Expenditure Management System in 1977 (see below), however, it was placed within the Economic Development envelope. The installation of two Ministries of State (for Social Development and for Economic Development) to advise the respective Policy Committees of Cabinet, meant that the need for its advice was somewhat diminished and its own placement attenuated its ties and influence·in the medical and social sciences areas. Consequently, it began to concern itself more with advising in growth areas of perceived economic importance, such as biotechnology, leaving the advising on programs of agencies in the Social Development envelope, which includes the Medical Research Council (MRC) and the Department of National Health and Welfare (NHW), more and more to the Ministry of State for Social Development. At the time of writing (pending the 1984 elections), the latter agency has been disbanded.

One major recommendation of the Senate Special Committee was that the government should establish a comprehensive science policy which would lead to harnessing the power of science to the achievement of national goals. Another was that the organisation of various federal agencies or scientific programs should be changed to allow better co-ordination and improve their effectiveness.

After assessing the practicality of these recommendations, it was realised that the idea of a comprehensive science policy is valid only at a level of great generality; consequently, the government announced, some ten years ago, its endorsement of a set of principles or science policies, including some for science, and some for the use of science. The latter include principles relating to the use of scientific approaches in the formation of public policy.

In its policies for science, the government recognises a federal responsibility to ensure the continued advancement of knowledge, especially in areas of direct importance to Canada, to maintain a scientific capability in Canada across all disciplines and to ensure a research training capacity to meet the continuing needs for research-trained manpower in all sectors of the economy. These goals are met, at present, largely through Canadian universities and the federal agencies charged with the basic responsibility for these commitments are the three granting Research Councils: the MRC, the Natural Sciences and Engineering Research Council (NSERC) and the Social Sciences and Humanities Research Council (SSHRC).

In its policies for the use of science, the government recognises a federal responsibility to develop the scientific knowledge needed to execute, or improve the execution of, its constitutionally-based functions. This goal is met both through the conduct of research in federal laboratories and through the acquisition of research results from other performers, both in Canada and abroad. Understandably, the knowledge needed will be most valuable if it is based on evidence generated within the Canadian context.

The government also recognises that scientific knowledge is not the only element that enters into

the execution of its constitutionally-based functions. We all know, for example, that fish-stocks
would be much better-protected if catches were kept
well below their present limits. However, the
livelihoods of many people would be threatened by
such a move and there are, thus, limits to the
extent to which scientific knowledge can be applied
in public policy. Nevertheless, the government
does believe that decisions should be informed by
the best scientifically-valid information possible
and should be taken using appropriate and scientifically sound procedures.

These, then, are the elements of 'science
policy' as it is understood by the federal government.

**Federal Mechanisms for the Implementation of Sci-
ence Policy**
As was mentioned above, a second recommendation of
the Senate Special Committee on Science Policy was
that the organisation of various federal agencies
or scientific programs should be changed to allow
better co-ordination and improved effectiveness.
Although the exact structure recommended by the
Senate Committee was not adopted, the principle of
reorganising the agencies responsible for maintaining research capability in Canada was accepted. In
a reorganisation implemented in 1977, the function
of supporting research in the social sciences and
humanities was assigned to the newly created SSHRC;
the Canada Council retained responsibility only for
the support and promotion of the fine and perform-
ing arts. Similarly, the external research-support
functions of the NRC were assigned to another new
Council, the NSERC; the NRC retained responsibility
only for its laboratories, the Canadian Institute
for Scientific and Technical Information and some
related functions. These changes gave the new
Councils the ability to concentrate on their single
responsibility of promoting and supporting research
- a function that was sometimes subordinated, by
the older Councils, to their other responsibilities.

The Medical Research Council remained un-
changed, except that a former restriction on supporting and promoting research in 'public health'
was removed. Through the three Councils, the
advancement of knowledge in all fields and the
maintenance of research-training capacity and
overall research capability in Canada was to be
ensured. Their activities are to be co-ordinated

through an Inter-Council Coordinating Committee, chaired by the Secretary of MOSST.

There is, of course, nothing to prevent the integration of principles relating to the support of science with those relating to the use of science. Recognising the need to advance knowledge and develop research capacity in areas of national concern, the government, in implementing the reorganisation of the granting Councils, has charged them to augment the traditional objectives (of ensuring excellence in research, promoting the general advancement of knowledge and maintaining a research-training capability in Canadian universities) with new objectives. These included developing a regional balance in research capacity, encouraging the selective concentration of research, facilitating multi-disciplinary research and promoting research that has the potential of contributing to national objectives. Relating these new emphases in policies in support of science to policies and programs designed to promote the use of science, the government announced in June, 1978 measures designed to stimulate research and development in Canada, particularly by Canadian industry. It hoped to increase the proportion of Gross National Product (GNP) spent on research and development (R & D) from 0.9 per cent in 1977 to 1.5 per cent by 1982.[3] For reasons which need not concern us here, industry has, for decades, been the performance sector most in need of stimulation in Canada. Among the government measures were some designed to induce small and medium-sized Canadian industries to embark upon research and development programs, but special increases were given to the three granting councils to promote research in areas of national concern. The Councils were encouraged to design new ways to facilitate the transfer of new knowledge from the universities where it is generated to the users where it will be applied. One means to do this is to encourage the flow of research-trained manpower into the user sphere, rather than supporting further expansion of research in the academic sector.

HEALTH SCIENCE POLICY

Health science policy, as such, has not been the object of such vigorous and open debate as was the case for science policy. Nor has it been the object of explicit policy development, at least at the federal level. Nevertheless, there has been

debate which surfaces at times, although the focus
of the debate tends to shift. For example, when
cutbacks in federal funds for all research were
proposed in the mid-70's, medical research, through
the aegis of MRC, argued for and won special consideration not accorded to research sponsored by
the other two granting Councils. In another instance, occurring about the same time, the question
of funding for non-medical health research was
raised, resulting in the formation of the departmental program known as the National Health Research and Development Program (NHRDP).

The debate in Canada tends to centre on the
relative merits of, and hence appropriate funding
levels for, medical research as opposed to other
health research. The former is quite unambiguously
equated to fundamental research in biochemistry,
physiology, genetics, pharmacology and other medical sciences, while the latter is variously identified as 'health care research', 'public health
research', or 'applied health research'. (Clinical
research, although 'applied', tends to be more
frequently associated with medical research than
with applied health research and its appropriate
share of funding debated within the context of
medical research rather than in opposition to it.)
Sometimes the distinction is drawn between 'curative' and 'preventive' research, with medical
science identified with the former or a disease-ori-
ented approach to health, and other disciplines
such as sociology, psychology and education identified with the latter or a health-promotional approach. Since 'public health' is not usually
equated with either 'health care' or 'health promotion', the opponents in the debate are not nearly
so unambiguously identifiable and seldom present a
unified voice to plead their cause vis-a-vis medical research. (Public health research concerns
itself with environmental factors affecting human
health and draws largely on a wide range of disciplines in the natural sciences, including, among
many others, toxicology, nutritional sciences,
bio-engineering and epidemiology; it relies heavily
on analysis of statistical data and forms the basis
for disease control and regulation of other environmental health hazards. Health care research, on
the other hand, concerns itself with the organisation and delivery of health care and draws on
possibly a wider range of disciplines which includes many of the social and administrative sciences.) Depending on which of these 'other' health
researches one wishes to promote, the contrast is

drawn between funding for (bio-)medical research, which is always high, and funding for the other, which is always low.

This debate underlay the establishment, in 1976, of the NHRDP whose founders negotiated a still-honoured agreement with MRC concerning their respective fields of support which were defined more or less as 'medical' and 'public health' research as explained above. The NHRDP, at the time, thus acquired a distinct 'population' or epidemiological flavour, even though a significant argument used in securing funds pointed to the growing need for research in health care delivery -- a reaction to the emerging and rapid escalation in health care costs for about half of which the federal government was reimbursing the provinces. An early emphasis of the program was to increase the supply of researchers competent in the area of health care delivery; to this end the NHRDP supported a series of 'Health Care Evaluation Seminars' which were designed to introduce research concepts and methodologies to health care practitioners. A significant outcome was to stimulate and, to the extent possible, satisfy an appetite for research among nurses. Research training was also supported through awards for graduate study in research, many of which were also made to nurses.

One might wish to note that various bodies, such as the World Health Organization, have called for a broader definition of health than merely the absence of disease and would include in 'health research' investigations related to such matters as the self-actualisation of women in male-dominated societies. Investigations of this kind would involve disciplines not usually thought of as health-related, including political science and economics as well as anthropology.

Because medical research advocates can point to resounding successes in the field and because they can also speak from a position of influence in society, bio-medical research continues to command both the bulk of popular support and the major share of federal health research funds. The present managers of the NHRDP have had greater success in competing for federal funds by stressing the relevance to the mission of the Department, NHW, of the research supported by the program, and by showing the usefulness of the research findings, than was possible when the arguments focused on the general need to develop research and research capability in non-medical health related fields such as epidemiology and health care. MRC, on the other hand, has defended its position as the guardian of fundamental research in danger of being lost in a sea of applied research supported by provincial governments, voluntary agencies and the mission-oriented Department. The question of federal support for research in health care delivery and in health$_4$ education within the formal educational system^4 then became less contentious because expenditure-dependent cost-sharing arrangements had been replaced by expenditure-dependent 'established program financing'.^{5} However, the question had resurfaced by 1984 and is currently being hotly debated within the context of changes to be negotiated further to the declaration of the Canada Health Act.

In short, federal health science policy may be said to be a commitment to support both fundamental and applied medical research in universities through the granting Councils, most particularly the MRC, as part of its general support for university research, and to support health research, wherever performed, that is related to various statutory obligations and departmental missions. This can be seen as a variant of the general science policy discussed earlier.

Other Health Science Policies

Commenting on health science policy at the provincial and voluntary agency level is, perhaps, somewhat hazardous but it seems safe to say that the provinces are motivated to promote research that promises to assist them in the containment of health care costs as well as research that enjoys popular support. Medical research, to find causes and cures, and clinical research, to test treatments and procedures, particularly research on major contributors to the 'health care burden' (cancers, heart disease, chronic and respiratory ailments) are primary recipients of provincial funds. By appealing simultaneously to popular support for medical research and popular desire to get 'something for nothing', several provinces have managed not only to obtain funds for medical research but also to provide themselves with some additional revenues by promoting their lotteries as a source of medical research funds. By funding medical research, the provincial governments gain popular support. Provincial health science policy, then, is probably a subset of provincial science policy that seeks to improve the provincial economy, either by promoting the production of goods and services or by reducing government expenditures.

Voluntary agencies, on the other hand, are usually associations of people who are either victims or relatives and friends of victims of specific ailments. Usually as a part of a broader program to provide services to the victims and their families, they are motivated to find cures or palliation for these ailments.

Thus, within the totality of funding for health research, in its broad sense, it can be seen that interest in promoting research in health care (and, within this, nursing research) now resides primarily with the provincial governments, apart from the general interest in supporting university research that is a federal commitment expressed through the three granting Councils. Where health care delivery is a federal responsibility and nurses and nursing are important agents for its execution -- for example, in nursing stations on Indian reservations and in the North, there is or ought to be interest at the federal level in sponsoring relevant research and in training and developing nurse researchers.

One recent development, however, that might affect the focus of various interests in health research is the coming into force in April, 1984, of the Canada Health Act. This Act is designed to consolidate the gains that Canadians have made in establishing a national system of publicly insured health care services in which the principles of accessibility, comprehensiveness, universality and portability are protected from the erosion that occurs when financial barriers such as extra-billing, user fees or premium charges, or other barriers such as excessive residency requirements are imposed by various jurisdictions within the system.

The new Act removes the policy and definitional concerns of health insurance -- the purview of Ministers of Health -- from the Federal-Provincial Fiscal Arrangements and Established Programs Financing Act, 1977 (the EPF Act), leaving questions of financing both health insurance and post-secondary education to be negotiated under the latter act by Ministers of Finance. (These fiscal arrangements are due to be re-negotiated in 1987.) The new Act has the rather limited objectives of clarifying the rules under which the federal government will assist the provinces in providing health services and of allowing the federal government greater flexibility in enforcing the rules by permitting the partial withholding of payments. (Under the EPF Act, only total withholding of payments was possible, a penalty that had never been imposed even though there had been breaches of the accessibility condition by some provinces as it was deemed to be too severe a sanction.)

By defining 'health care practitioner', 'insured services', 'medical services', 'comprehensiveness', of services and 'necessary' services as being, in essence, whatever the provinces, through their licensing and regulatory laws and actions, define them to be, the Canada Health Act also places the onus clearly on the provinces to decide what is to be the future role of nurses, optometrists, chiropractors and other health practitioners in the Canadian health care system.

Although the new Act has the rather limited objectives just mentioned, it may prove to have a wider and more important effect. Weller and Manga (1983, pp. 223-246) have very well described the evolution of health policy in Canada during the last forty years. They show how, first, shared-cost public insurance was substituted for the prior 'laissez-faire' that left both health care delivery and health insurance in the private realm. Although this had the very desirable effect of bringing equity into the health care system, it also initiated and entrenched the politicisation of health care and the centrality of the hospital in the system. Then the EPF fiscal arrangements were substituted for the preceding cost-shared arrangements, further heightening the subordination of the substantive issues of the balance between curative and preventive medicine, the need for community health centres and the need for cheaper physician substitutes to the constitutional, financial and inter-governmental aspects of health policy. The new Canada Health Act, by opening the door to a redefinition of what constitute insured services, health care practitioners and medical services and thus de-emphasising the constitutional and inter-governmental aspects and by separating health policy negotiations from fiscal negotiations, may also be paving the way to refocusing health policy on the substantive issues. Depending on these developments, the interests in health care research may vary accordingly.

We turn now to give an overview of health research funding and a final glimpse of the current place of nursing research within that picture.

HEALTH RESEARCH FUNDING

Growth of Programs and Policy Mechanisms

Starting at the federal level, we find the MRC which, since its birth as part of the NRC, has been the major source of funds for health-related research. Its budget for supporting and developing the medical research component of health research in Canada grew from about $7 million in 1964-65 to $37 million in 1972-73 and to approximately $135 million in 1983-84. Although it no longer has responsibility for research in the social sciences and humanities, the Canada Council still administers bequests from the Killam family which provide income for inter- or cross-disciplinary research, including health research. That fund has provided about $1 million annually for scholarships, fellowships and research associateships in the fields of science, engineering and medicine. A former requirement to demonstrate a link between the disciplines involved and some areas of social sciences and humanities had been dropped by the mid-seventies.

As noted earlier, the Councils are not the only federal agencies involved with health research. The federal Laboratory of Hygiene was established in 1913; its activities were gradually expanded and the Laboratory itself was the nucleus for what is presently the Health Protection Branch of NHW. From the inception of the Laboratory, research was and still remains an important activity of the Branch, serving as the base for the monitoring and regulatory functions associated with administering various Acts, for example, the Food and Drugs, Narcotics Control and Hazardous Products Acts, and also as the base for carrying out responsibilities shared with other federal departments, such as implementing the Clean Air, Environmental Contaminants and Clean Water Acts. By the early '80s, this intramural element of health-related research in Canada was supported by expenditures of approximately $35 million annually.

An extramural research support component was added by the Department in 1948, in the form of the Public Health Research Grant -- an element of a broader program of General Health Grants designed to assist the provinces in building their health care delivery systems. This particular Grant was supplemented in 1972 by the National Health Grant, which was intended to support extramural research needed in fulfilling other Departmental responsibilities, for example the provision of health

services to special populations such as Indians and
residents of the northern Territories, the provision of medical services to public servants and on
board coast guard vessels, the examination and
treatment of immigrants, or the maintenance of
international quarantines and the surveillance of
diseases that may be imported from abroad. In
1976, the Public Health Research Grant and the
National Health Grant were amalgamated to form the
NHRDP. It is designed to encourage and support
extramural research related to Departmental responsibilities and, when necessary, to support and
develop an extramural research capacity capable of
responding to the Department's research requirements. In addition to the NHRDP, the Department
has, from time to time, set up special research-sup-
porting programs focused on particular problems of
special significance. Examples of such programs
include those aimed at supporting research on drug
abuse, fitness and amateur sport and civil aviation
medicine. By the middle '70s, these programs
supported annually nearly $20 million worth of
research, development and related scientific activities, with an additional $2 million allotted to
research in two other social service-related grants
programs that impinge on health, that is, Welfare
Grants and Family Planning Grants programs. Since
that time, all but the civil aviation medicine
research program have been integrated into either
the NHRDP or the Welfare Grants program.

While the federal government was thus developing policies and programs supporting both health
research and the development of health research
capability in Canada, the provinces were also
extending their interests beyond the provision of
health services to include research related to
health and health care. Doubtless much of the
impetus came from the rapidly rising costs of
health services and a desire to find ways to contain them but it probably was also augmented by the
provinces' growing interest in science policy and
research in general: science advisory bodies were
established in several provinces and a federal-provincial Canadian Committee on Financing University
Research was set up in 1975 (and later forgotten).

Various provincial mechanisms were established
to advise on or fund health research. In the late
'70s, provincial deputy ministers of health set up
an inter-provincial committee to examine priorities
for health research and help to co-ordinate various
research efforts. Its point of departure was the
1977 report of the Ontario Council of Health,

addressed to health research priorities for that province. One should also mention the Inter-Agency Health Research Coordinating Group which meets about every two years to exchange information on current funding of health research and on related policies. It is composed of representatives of the major funding agencies, including those of the federal and provincial governments and voluntary organisations.

Funding of Health Research

In 1978, federal funding of health research and related scientific activities totalled about $110 million -- $27 million spent intramurally by NHW, and $83 million spent extramurally -- $20 million by NHW and $63 million by MRC. By 1983, these expenditures had risen to a total of about $190 million ($35 million intramurally and $20 million extramurally by the Department and $135 million by the MRC.)

We have not been able to estimate how much the provinces might spend intramurally in the various health ministries; we do know that by the late '70s Ontario was spending about $15 million directly on research, including support of Foundations for Heart, Mental Health, Addiction Research, and Cancer Treatment Research, Wintario grants and health research grants and scholarships; Quebec was spending about $12 million in direct support of hospital and clinical investigations and to increase the number of health researchers through training as well as supporting newly-trained researchers; and Alberta, with income from its Heritage Fund, made a significant investment in basic medical research and gave $10 million to its hospitals to develop a comprehensive program of research in cancer and heart disease, including prevention, treatment and rehabilitation. About the same time, British Columbia, through its B.C. Health Care Research Foundation, funded from the Western Express Lottery, spent some $2.7 million in support of health care research. By 1983, direct support for health research at the provincial level exceeded $60 million annually. Assuming that hidden costs of research are approximately equal to direct costs, the provinces are also providing as much as $325 million indirectly, in the form of principal investigator salaries, facilities and overheads on health research carried out in their universities and hospitals.

To the picture should be added about $50 million provided by voluntary organisations, such as the National Cancer Institute, the Canadian Heart Foundation and the Cerebral Palsy Association and about $50 million spent on health research by Canadian industry, primarily by the pharmaceutical industry.

In all, some $640 million is being spent annually on medical and health research and related scientific activities (such as research training, testing and standardisation, and scientific data collection) in Canada: a little less than one-third of this by the federal government; a little over one-half directly and indirectly by the provinces; and the balance by industry and voluntary organisations.

We have deliberately chosen to include an estimation of the indirect costs of research in our discussion, even though the assumption in the estimate may be questioned. (Some claim indirect costs run about 50 cents on the research dollar; others claim they are four times that amount.) We have done so because there are those who wish to compare our health research effort here in Canada with that of other countries where funding practices are very different. In the US, for example, research grants from the National Institutes of Health include allowances for principal investigators' salaries as well as indirect costs and often provide for consultation at high per diem rates.

Insofar as nursing research is concerned, almost no MRC funding has been given to nurses, as is the case to date with SSHRC. It is widely recognised that NHRDP has played the key role in funding nursing research, albeit within the context of its broadly cast extramural funding program aimed at responding to NHW's research requirements rather than at responding to the needs of nursing research *per se*. Statistics indicate that in 1976-77, out of expenditures totalling $8.2 million, it supported 17 projects in nursing entailing expenditures of about $800,000; in 1977-78, out of expenditures totalling $10.6 million, it supported 19 projects costing $1.4 million. Reflecting the reality, noted earlier, of having to show the departmental relevance of the research it supports in order to secure funds, research related to public health as opposed to research related to health care delivery has been gaining a larger and larger share of NHRDP funds. This may have no bearing, however, on the fact that in 1983-84 there were only 16 projects in nursing research,

commanding only $300,000 out of the total budget of
$16.1 million. The fact of the matter is that the
content of nursing research has shifted from concern with demonstrations of expanded roles for
nurses to concern with experimental designs in
assessing treatment outcomes. The latter type of
research is much less expensive. The NHRDP has
also given considerable support to national nursing
research conferences and has often funded as many
as ten nurses per year through its Student Fellowship program.

We now turn to an analysis of the processes by
which decisions are made about allocating funds to
federal level research, including health care
research.

POLICY AND EXPENDITURE MANAGEMENT SYSTEM

Probably the most significant development affecting
science policy and the funding of health research
within the last ten years has been the introduction
of a new policy and expenditure management system
by the Federal government. Put simply, the old
method of planning and forecasting budget requirements was to consider programs individually, allowing increments 'on demand' whenever justifications
were sufficiently convincing, and then adding them
all up to produce a total budget. This has been
replaced by planning and budgeting within the
framework of anticipated resources. In this new
system, five-year forecasts are used to plan both
resources and expenditures, thus providing both the
basis and the need to order government priorities.
In principle, to start new programs or increase
expenditures in existing ones means reducing or
eliminating allocations to others.

At present, Ministers responsible for government departments or agencies belong to one of four
Cabinet Committees -- Economic Development, Social
Development, Foreign Policy and Defense, and Government Operations. Secretariat support for the
first two committees was, until very recently,
provided by a Ministry of State -- for Economic and
Regional development and for Social Development,
respectively -- while Secretariat services for the
other two were provided by the Privy Council Office
(PCO). (At least for the time being, all four are
now served by the PCO. The new government may
decide to change this and may even decide to change
the whole system.) The Ministers' departments and
agencies are included in a corresponding budgetary

envelope. The allocation to each envelope is made
by the most senior Cabinet Committee -- Priorities
and Planning; the annual adjustments reflect the
government's currently anticipated revenues, expenditures on statutory programs such as Unemployment
Insurance and Family Allowances, and acceptable
levels of deficit. These allocations are shown in
the 'Main Estimates' tabled each year in the House
of Commons, about the end of February. Because it
is always desirable to have the flexibility to
respond to evolving situations, 'reserves' have
been created within each envelope, either through
reduction or elimination of low-priority programs,
as is the case in the Social Development envelope,
or through the allocation of money earmarked for
specific purposes, as in the case of the 'energy
reserve' in the Economic Development envelope.
Before the budget year begins, Ministers of a given
envelope put forward proposals to be considered for
funding from its reserve; they then meet at intervals during the budget year and decide how much of
the reserve will be spent and for what purposes.
Usually, this is done by reviewing the arguments
put forward by the proposing Minister and comments
provided by their own advisors and by the Ministry
of State or PCO group that advises on both the
present and continuing implications of the proposal
in the context of the envelope as well as on its
merits, Ministers decide which proposals to accept
and the budgetary allocations to be made. Part of
the input to this decision-making process is an
overview of the proposals which are still waiting
to be considered.

This system of management has obvious implications for both science policy and the federal
funding of health research, whether intramural or
extramural. Science policy, to influence budgetary
allocations, must be integral to the process of
setting overall government priorities; health
research, to make gains or even to hold its own in
the competition for funds, must state its objectives or demonstrate its benefits in terms that can
be matched to these priorities. Thus, if science
policy is to remain influential (for example, in
sustaining the thrust to increase Canadian investments in research and other scientific activities),
it will do so in proportion as science shows itself
able to lead to economic or social benefits; if
health research is to keep its share of an envelope's resources, it must convince everyone that it
is as important as, let us say, social programs
such as old age pensions. This is no easy task,

given the disparity in visible benefit from expenditures made on scientific programs (which may reach a conclusion only in several years' time and then take additional years to have the results incorporated into products or practices) versus expenditures on programs aimed at assisting individuals disadvantaged by present circumstances. The possibility of adding a new program or program thrust is only as great as the possibility of dropping something else.

This system of management means, too, that once a fiscal year has begun, any marginal reallocations of funds will most likely occur within a 'vote' -- the individual allotment made to specific 'programs' that are identified in the government budget and to which funds are voted by Parliament in the process of approving the budget. (A given department may administer several 'votes', as is the case with NHW, or may administer only one, as is the case with the MRC.) This is because money released from any given 'vote' is automatically placed in the envelope's reserve, thereby removing it from the control of a single Minister; there is no guarantee that it will be reallocated to another vote within that Minister's control.

In practical terms, these constraints mean that the planning horizon has been pushed farther out, since the general thrust of envelope adjustments is determined three or four years in advance of the current fiscal year, thus allowing appropriate adjustments to be made within them. Where statutory limitations exist, such as a requirement to give advance notice of a change in federal-provincial fiscal transfer arrangement, such as that governing the Established Program Financing, flexibility in planning is correspondingly reduced.

A second development worthy of note is that the government's desire for greater 'relevance' in the programs of the three granting Research Councils -- MRC, NSERC, and SSHRC -- expressed in the new goals that were set for them in 1976 (see Science Policy, above), have gradually had a discernible effect on their programs. Although all the Councils play a largely reactive role, responding with the bulk of their funds to proposals for research on topics freely chosen by university scientists and scholars, they have clearly moved toward leading the scientific community in areas of national and regional concern, that is, moving toward strategic programming.

NSERC was first to respond with a five year plan that was acceptable, in principle, to the

Cabinet. This plan was based on forecasts of scientific manpower production in the natural sciences by Canadian universities, on analysis of the impact of other science policy thrusts -- primarily the programs designed to stimulate industrial R&D -- for scientific manpower in appropriate fields, and on the identification of major strategic areas where R&D should be able to make important contributions to the benefit of Canadians in the relatively near future. Thus, the plan incorporated new programs of scholarships and fellowships, oriented toward industrial research and project support in the strategic areas of energy, environmental toxicology, oceans, communications and agriculture/food. Projects in these areas command approximately 12 percent of the total budget, while manpower programs command approximately 6 percent.

SSHRC was next to have its five year plan approved, in principle, by Cabinet. In this plan, Canadian Studies -- broadly defined to include research on Canadian economic, social and cultural features, whether in a historical, dynamic or comparative sense -- will gradually command a greater share of the budget, while the strategic areas of population aging and professional studies, including business management, law and education, will be given special encouragement within the Canadian Studies program. The latest five year plans of both NSERC and SSHRC are currently under budgetary review.

MRC put forward its first five year plan in 1983. For the Council, a most significant event was the loss, in 1977, of its founding President, Dr G. Malcolm Brown, whose vision had shaped its programs for nearly twenty years. Of his successors, the one who appears to have been most actively seeking to bring new ideas into the Council's programs is the current President, Dr Pierre Bois. Under his guidance, the Council has held two retreats (in October, 1981 and April, 1982) to examine the changing milieu of the Council's operations and its role as a federal agency, its interactions with the academic community and the needs for and means of identifying priorities and implementing them.

The three Council Presidents, collectively, have seen the need for improving the interactions among their programs. Although there has been for years a formal link between them -- the Tri-Council Coordinating Committee until 1977, followed by the Inter-Council Coordinating Committee -- the matters considered have tended to be administrative rather than substantive. Thus there have been co-ordination of matters such as stipends for scholars and fellows and agreement on matters such as how to distribute proposals in disciplines that span all three Councils, in particular, mathematics and psychology. However, it is only recently that there seems to have developed a will to co-ordinate interdisciplinary research or to try to accommodate areas of research or scholarship that do not fit neatly into the natural or life sciences on the one hand or the social sciences on the other. These developments would appear to be commodious for nursing research which is so broad in scope that it does not fit neatly into any one program. Thus, it is hoped that in its current reexamination of its role in research funding, the federal government will give close attention to the case for making definitive provision for the funding of nursing research.

NOTES

1. For fuller treatment of the evolution of and inputs to science policy in Canada, see Chapter 3, sections B, C and D, of the Government of Canada Background Report to the O.E.C.D. Examiners, for the O.E.C.D. Review of Education Policy: Canada, 1974.

2. The first three volumes contained its findings and recommendations.

3. The target year was later pushed back to 1985; by 1982, Gross Expenditures on R&D had reached 1.3 percent of GNP but the level has since fallen to 1.2 percent in 1984, due to the general recession.

4. Except for specific pockets of federal responsibility, such as on Indian reservations and for the armed forces, health care delivery and education are both areas of provincial responsibility.

5. Under the new arrangements, federal payments to the provinces are made on a per capita basis, using an escalation factor applied to the national average expenditure in a certain base year. This means that federal payments are made without regard to a given province's

current expenditures on insured health services and federal interest in cost-containment (as well as in research supportive of that goal) is thereby diminished.

REFERENCES

Weller, G.R., and Manga, P. (1983). The development of health policy in Canada. In *The Politics of Canadian Public Policy*, M.M. Atkinson and M.A. Chandler (Eds.), University of Toronto Press, Toronto, pp. 223-246.

Chapter Six

STRUCTURE AND FUNDING OF NURSING RESEARCH IN CANADA

Janet C. Kerr

THE GROWTH OF GRADUATE EDUCATION AND RESEARCH

Because most Canadian universities secured considerable numbers of their faculty members from British
institutions prior to World War I, the influence of
British thinking may be seen in the acceptance of
the notion of: 'the primacy of undergraduate education, and on the secondary and supplementary place
of graduate studies and research' (Bonneau and
Corry, 1972, p. 18). However, between 1920 and 1940
the number of full-time students enrolled in graduate programs in Canadian universities rose to almost
four times the original figure of 423, and the
percentage of total enrollment accounted for by
graduate students increased from 1.8% to 4.3%
(Harris, 1975, p. 428). During this period of time
influences from the United States in the Germanic
tradition began to be felt as universities awarded
faculty appointments to Canadian products of the
graduate schools of the United States (Bonneau and
Corry, 1972, p. 18). This was particularly notice-
able at Toronto and McGill, which: 'established
graduate schools and gave a high rating to research'
(Bonneau and Corry, 1972, p. 18). The impact of the
American influences became significant following
World War II and increased until: 'About 1960, they
became pervasive' (Bonneau and Corry, 1972, p. 18).
Further, this period saw 'spectacular expansion' of
graduate studies in the sciences and considerable
pressure for continued development: 'There is no
point in skimping on graduate work and research when
these form one of the key factors in our continued
existence as an independent nation' (Spinks, 1962,
pp. 32-38).

The expansion referred to was due primarily to the stimulus to graduate work provided by the National Research Council, under the aegis of which financial support to Canadian universities had increased thirty-fold since 1939 to 10.5 million in 1960-61 (Harris, 1975, p. 553). Progress in the humanities and social sciences lagged behind that in the sciences however, and special efforts were required to restore the balance. One of the resolutions passed by the National Conference of Canadian Universities at its 1944 meeting was as follows:

> Resolved that the Conference direct the attention of the Universities and the Governments concerned to the generally inadequate state of graduate work in the humanities and the social sciences in Canadian universities and to the necessity of restoring and building it up to the level of the Master's degree and thereby giving life to undergraduate instruction and to the teaching profession in secondary and other schools (National Conference of Canadian Universities, 1944, p. 27).

Basic to the concerns was the knowledge that there would need to be a great infusion of resources to meet the needs of the veterans who would be returning following demobilization in view of the depleted ranks of academic staff brought about by the war effort. Accordingly the Social Science Research Council and the Humanities Research Council initiated a program of fellowships in 1946 and 1947 respectively with funds provided by the Carnegie Corporation of New York and the Rockefeller Foundation (Harris, 1975, p. 559). With the creation of the Canada Council in 1957, support was offered at both master's and doctoral levels. For example, in 1960-61 this agency granted 221 fellowships involving an aggregate expenditure of $350,000 (Harris, 1975, p. 559). Graduate studies in professional fields also began to open up in the postwar period and developed with support from the granting councils along with the rapid escalation in the size of the graduate education enterprise taking place in the sciences.

Federal Support for Research
The federal government first recognized a need for improved research and development because of the war effort, and formed the National Research Council (NRC) in 1916. Since that time its role has been

focused upon 'undertaking, assisting and promoting scientific and industrial research in Canada' in certain specified areas (Secretary of State, 1975, p. 2). In 1975-76 there were three Councils which were responsible for funding university-based research: the Medical Research Council (MRC) which was formed in 1939 and the Canada Council, formed in 1957 to support research in the humanities and social sciences, as well as NRC. There are, in addition, other agencies and departments of the federal government which are involved in granting smaller amounts of support to research. One of these, Health and Welfare Canada, has particular importance for the nursing profession in terms of research support under the National Health Research and Development Program (NHRDP).

Three categories of federal research support provide funds in the form of research grants, research fellowships and auxiliary grants, the latter providing only indirect support for research. Funds may be awarded directly to faculty members and/or institutions: 'to assist them in the performance of projects initiated and controlled by the grant recipients' (Secretary of State, 1975, p. 35). Fellowships, on the other hand, are funds which are channelled directly to faculty members for research activities which have the development of research competence as their primary objective. In 1972-73 spending had reached a level of 121 million with NRC responsible for 46.75% of this total, MRC for 28.05% and the Canada Council for 6.78%. Health and Welfare Canada, under the NHRDP, was responsible for 4.36% of the funds awarded (Secretary of State, 1975). This level of spending represented a rise from 118 million in 1969-70, a considerable increase from the almost negligible sums that were available prior to 1951 when the Massey Commission declared that research support was one of the: 'areas for which federal assistance was not only constitutionally permissable but socially necessary' (Peitchinis, 1971, p. 33).

However, from 1971-1974 federal research funding in Canada experienced a period of no growth, and in December, 1975, the funds of the MRC were temporarily frozen with the result that research teams across the country had to curtail or discontinue their research activities, leaving all in a state of limbo. The 'hard line' taken by the federal government towards medical research had been vigourously denounced by the medical community:

> Those who downplay research show little incli-
> nation to give up its practical benefits. Only
> the cost is shunned, not the fruits. If
> Canadians want the high quality of health care
> they deserve, they must be prepared to pay for
> it. And a reasonable tab for medical research
> must remain prominently displayed on the
> invoice (Osmond, 1976, p. 10).

Thus the course for the future in terms of federal
research policy remains highly uncertain. Whether
or not the medical community will be successful in
its efforts to improve the situation and regain
support for the research endeavor is unknown. Also
unknown is the question of whether or not the
research budgets of other Councils, agencies and
departments will be subjected to similar treatment,
and the priority that will be given to research in a
period of time when the country is suffering from
the effects of general economic instability.

Recent and interesting developments which may
eventually have some impact on federal funding for
health research centre around provincial research
funding activities. In the province of Ontario a
lottery has been introduced, the proceeds of which
are targeted for health research, and in Alberta in
1980 the provincial government created the Alberta
Heritage Foundation for Medical Research (AHFMR), a
research granting agency, by allocating 300 million
dollars from the Heritage Savings Trust Fund. The
interest on this principal was targeted to the
support of medical research activities. Then, in
1982, the Alberta Government established the Alberta
Foundation for Nursing Research (AFNR) by ministeri-
al order, for the support of nursing research
activities. One million dollars was granted to the
Foundation to be awarded to nurse researchers whose
projects were recommended for approval over a period
of five years. The first chairman of AFNR appointed
by the Alberta Government was Dr. Shirley M.
Stinson, a vigorous proponent of the need for
greater financial support for nursing research. In
relation to both of the latter funds, it can be said
that involvement in the financing of health research
on the part of a provincial government represents a
rare, unique and welcome intervention into the
financing of research activities.

Building the Foundation for Nursing Research
Growth of research activity in nursing has occurred
gradually as a consequence of a slowly increasing

pool of nurses with preparation for undertaking research projects. Such development goes hand in hand with, and is a necessary condition for, the establishment of graduate education in nursing, for the bulk of the research in any field takes place in university settings and the teaching of research methods is an important facet of graduate education. Since the development of graduate education in nursing has only recently become an identifiable thrust, that is, in the past 25 years, this has had its effect upon nursing research activities. Master's degree programs are now established in sufficient numbers to ensure availability on a wider scale to prospective students, but doctoral programs are still on the horizon in Canada. The approval of new programs on the part of universities is, at the best of times, let alone times of entrenchment, unlikely without extensive evidence of substantial research activity in the particular school and of faculty qualifications at the doctoral level. This has been the 'catch-22' for nursing -- demonstrating research capability and productivity as well as faculty expertise in the absence of the availability of doctoral programs in nursing in Canada.

The unfolding of the entire range of university programs in nursing from baccalaureate through doctoral levels is a process which is well underway, but by no means nearing completion. Rationalizing the process rests on the view of the university as 'a social institution, the specific mission of which is the transmission and the advancement of higher learning.' Bonneau and Corry describe the association between teaching and research as a natural one, albeit complex, and elaborate. 'Some kinds of research, and some features of the research enterprise, are vital for good teaching: every university teacher should be involved in these kinds of features, and supported in them under the teaching budget' (Bonneau and Corry, 1972, p. 23).

At the conclusion of the sometimes stormy decade of the 60's, Canadian universities became engaged in responding to the challenges and issues raised. One criticism that was levelled at the institutions throughout that period of rapid growth and student unrest was that too much time and energy were being expended upon the research endeavour and too little upon identifying and encouraging excellence in teaching. It is somewhat curious that universities came under fire for supposedly being preoccupied with research at precisely the same period of time as the nursing profession was engaged in the difficult struggle to establish its first graduate programs. In the process of so doing, the need for development of its research potential was underscored. Symons has commented as follows: 'The slowness in developing graduate schools of nursing in Canada has, in turn, adversely effected [sic] the amount of research undertaken in this field. Little support has been available for publication, or for investigating problems in nursing health care of particular interest to Canadians' (Symons, 1975, p. 212).

In her delineation of the meaning of the concepts of professionalization and deprofessionalization, Stinson postulates that the development of the research function is a vital component of the former:

> Supplying professional services inheres in the principle that initiating research, training various kinds of research workers, and 'marketing' findings must not be left to the whims of chance and/or at the entire mercy of commercial interests. This means evolving not only intra-professional mechanisms for the development and application of substantive knowledge but articulating these devices with those of other professions and those of the broader society (Stinson, 1969, p. 167).

Although the need and concomitant timeliness of research in nursing has been recognised both within and without the profession, there have been problems in effecting change and it is likely that these will continue to present as stumbling blocks for some time to come. The social reality of the last quarter of the twentieth century is that limits to growth of universities have appeared in the form of greatly decreased numbers of learners entering the 18 to 22 year age group. This situation has occurred simultaneously with, at least in the early part of the period referred to, adverse world economic circumstances leading to shaky national economies, and subsequently to financial stringency in all public institutions. However slow the basic elements in research and graduate study in nursing though, there is little doubt that the process will continue, and Stinson asserts that successful delivery of nursing services to society will ultimately require: 'that three simultaneous processes be going on: (1) *accumulation* of the K-S [knowledge-skill] component, (2) *transmission* of it, and (3) *extension* of it, mainly through *systematic research*' (Stinson, 1969, pp. 156-157).

Concerted efforts to develop organisational support for nursing began in earnest in the early seventies, when attention had been drawn to the crucial nature of that support by Stinson:

A paradox of modern day research is that it is at once an intensely individual, personal endeavour, yet, if it is to be brought about, much less constitute benefits for society, it is immensely dependent upon organization - and highly complex organization at that (Stinson, 1977, p. 10).

The first national conference on nursing research in Canada was held in Ottawa in 1971 under the auspices of federal assistance under the National Health Research and Development Program. As this was a 'first' for the nursing profession in Canada, historical overviews were presented on the kinds of nursing research projects conducted over the years by governments and services agencies, the professional association and universities (Griffin, 1971; Imai, 1971; and Poole, 1971). These papers document the fact that although there has been a certain amount of activity over the years, the majority of studies have been undertaken since 1965, some of which were funded by a variety of sponsoring agencies. However, in relation to university-based projects, Griffin commented:

Funds for either faculty or graduate student research have not been obtained for many projects. Of those reported, only 22 faculty and 23 students indicated some sponsorship. A few respondents indicated funds had not been obtained 'yet' and doubtlessly the graduate students were indirectly funded for their research through funding all or part of the graduate education programs (Griffin, 1971, p. 96).

FUNDING FOR NURSING RESEARCH

The three primary areas for which external research support is sought include: (1) research projects, (2) research training, and (3) research facilities (Stinson, 1977, pp. 21-25). This discussion will be limited to the first two areas as they necessarily precede and condition the eventual development of the third. However, it should be noted that the first Centre for Nursing Research was established at

McGill University in 1971 with federal support from
Health and Welfare Canada. Until funding for
nursing became more readily available as an integral
part of the terms of reference of the National
Health Research and Development Program of Health
and Welfare Canada, there were few sources of funds
for either research projects or research training
other than the rather limited funds of the Canadian
Nurses Foundation and those, also limited, of the
private foundations and voluntary organisations.
Even the 1971 documentation provided by Griffin and
referred to above indicates that research funding
has not been secured for great numbers of projects,
even in the recent past. Further, the following
additional qualification should be noted:

> It must be underlined that, to date, as sub-
> stantial proportion of Canadian nursing re-
> search has been done by graduate students at
> their own expense, and by nursing faculty and
> health agency members, often on their own time,
> and on a non-funded basis. As such, direct
> cost figures give us only a hint of the time,
> equipment, supplies and publication costs of
> all the nursing research being done (Ibid., p.
> 22).

It is noteworthy that a variety of sources of
funding for research have been opening up for nurses
in various provinces over the past decade and a
half. Among these new sources of funding are the
Alberta Foundation for Nursing Research, the B.C.
Health Care Research Foundation, the Canadian Heart
Foundation, the Hospital for Sick Children Founda-
tion, the Kidney Foundation of Canada, the Ontario
Ministry of Health and the Saskatchewan Health
Research Board.

FEDERAL SUPPORT FOR RESEARCH PROJECTS IN NURSING

A review of federal research grants for projects
relating to health care between 1949 and 1963
indicated that no funding was awarded for research
projects in university schools of nursing (Defence
Research Board, 1963). Beginning in 1963, support
began to become available in progressively incremental amounts for research in nursing (see Table 6.1).
Although the funds documented in Table 6.1 were
reported to have been allocated for nursing research
between 1963 and 1968, funding for only one

investigation carried out by a nurse co-principal
investigator from a university school of nursing
could be identified from a review of lists of all
health sciences projects funded in those years
(Good, 1969, p. 21). The nurse co-principal investigator with project funding was H.M. Carpenter of
the University of Toronto, whose cooperative project
with an Eastshore-Leaside health unit investigator
received a federal grant of $7,100 (Defence Research
Board, 1967, p. 18). Notwithstanding the relatively
recent availability of research funds for nursing it
may be readily ascertained from a review of Table
6.1 that funding began to increase dramatically
after that period of time, until in 1975-76,
$572,005 was awarded for nursing research projects
in university schools of nursing.

Table 6.1

Research Project Grants to Nurses
from Federal Sources:
1964-1968 and 1972-1976

Year	Amount Awarded
1964-65	$11,300
1965-66	25,074
1966-67	27,414
1967-68	28,415
1972-73	148,497
1973-74	101,563
1974-75	152,031
1975-76	572,005

Federal support awarded for nursing research in
this year thus provided funding for fifteen research
projects under the direction of ten nurse-principal
investigators across the country. In 1974-75, the
$152,031 which was awarded to nurse-principal
investigators was distributed across ten projects
under the direction of eight investigators. The
increase in the level of federal support for nursing
research between 1974-75 and 1975-76 can be seen to
be a substantial 38%. There was an even greater
increase in funding from 1973-74 to 1974-75, with
$101,563 being awarded in the former year over five
projects and four principal investigators. The
increase between those two years amounts to 71.2%.
In relation to this latter figure, however, it
should be noted that there was a decline in funding

from the year 1972-73 to 1973-74, a fact which might account for the very substantial rise in the following year. The decline referred to represented a 46.2% drop in the level of funding for nursing research. Considered within the eleven-year time span reported in Table 6.1, federal allocations for nursing research projects have gone from a rather modest $11,300 in 1964-65 to the more sizeable figure of $572,000 in 1975-76. The greater part of this development in nursing research stimulated by federal funding has occurred under the auspices of the National Health Research and Development Program. Since 1971 five national conferences on nursing research have received federal funding under this program as well, and undoubtedly these have contributed in no small measure to the development of research skills amongst nurse researchers.

RESEARCH SUPPORTED BY UNIVERSITY SCHOOLS OF NURSING

Efforts were directed in the course of the data-gathering process towards documenting the research support reported by university schools of nursing. Table 6.2 reports the results of those efforts and documents the funds designated for nursing research expended by schools as reported by the individual universities. Although data were collected for the entire period of study, it was concluded that the most useful information was reported in the years of the last decade, because almost all of the earlier support designated as research funding was essentially private funding received for the development of new or innovative programs. Therefore Table 6.2 is limited to the period from 1965-66 to 1980-81.

The significant change in the size and extent of research enterprises in university schools of nursing over time may be seen in Table 6.2. From a very small endeavour in just a few schools, nursing research has become a more broadly-based and much better financed undertaking. Although the figures reported are aggregate sums which may include funds received from external granting agencies for program development, they nevertheless give some indication of 'the state of the art'. The figures reported for the University of British Columbia are exceptions to this general statement, however, as it can be seen that at that institution there is a distinction made between funding for research projects and those external grant funds expended for program development by designating the latter as special-purpose funds. Funds reported for Dalhousie University were

TABLE 2

Funds Expended for Nursing Research Reported by Canadian University Schools of Nursing, 1965-66 to 1980-81

	1980-81	1975-76		1970-71		1965-66	
	Assisted Research: Nursing	Assisted Research: Nursing	Percent of Total University Research Funds	Assisted Research: Nursing	Percent of Total University Research Funds	Assisted Research: Nursing	Percent of Total University Research Funds
University of British Columbia	13,074	104,333 385,296[a]	2.95%	19,805 10,373[a]	0.27%	1,519	0.03%
University of Alberta	0	18,366	0.14%	13,126	0.17%	b	b
University of Saskatchewan	7,135						
University of Manitoba	0	88,728	0.10%	0	0	b	b
University of Western Ontario	0	7,232	0.06%	6,711	0.10%	0	0
University of Toronto	89,070	171,574	0.58%	84,723	0.44%	12,091	b

TABLE 2 (continued)

	1980-81	1975-76		1970-71		1965-66	
	Assisted Research: Nursing	Assisted Research: Nursing	Percent of Total University Research Funds	Assisted Research: Nursing	Percent of Total University Research Funds	Assisted Research: Nursing	Percent of Total University Research Funds
McMaster University	101,517						
Universite de Montreal	0	61,363	0.32%	0	0	b	b
McGill University	61,663	170,892	0.81%	35,242	0.23%	b	b
Dalhousie University	0	0	0	92,606	2.69%	37,063	b

SOURCES: Financial statements, accountants' records and records of the schools of nursing of the above universities; Reference List of Health Science Research in Canada, 1980-81 (source for 1980-81 information).

[a]"Special purpose" funds refer to program development funds
[b]Information unavailable.

also entirely allocated for program costs, in this
case, of the Outpost Nursing program supported by
Health and Welfare Canada. It is a point of some
interest that all of the universities operating
graduate programs in 1980-81 are listed in Table 6.2
with the addition of one other university not yet
operating a graduate program and which reported
substantial research funding.

The information presented in Table 6.2 demonstrates that in the year 1965-66 the research
funding picture in schools of nursing was bleak
indeed. The $12,091 reported for the University of
Toronto resulted from the interest from endowment
funds, and while it may have been applied to research projects, it is more likely that it was
applied to support undergraduate instruction in the
School at that time. It may also be seen that
Kellogg funding for the development of the master's
program at the University of Western Ontario had
been exhausted by 1965-66. The largest external
grant of those schools reporting was to Dalhousie
University and, as noted above, these federal monies
were not used for research or graduate programming,
but for the operating support of a diploma program.
However, some gaps exist in the information obtained, and therefore it should be recognized that
Table 6.2 does not present a complete picture of the
year 1965-66.

In contrast to the meager support seen in
1965-66, in 1970-71 there would appear to have been
a marked increase in both the size of the support
being received by various schools and in the number
of schools securing assistance. The University of
Toronto graduate program supported by Kellogg funds
was established in that year and Table 6.2 shows
that external grant funds for nursing were becoming
responsible for a steadily increasing percentage of
the total research funding for that institution
moving from 0.14% in 1965-66 to 0.44% in 1970-71.
Again, in that year the Dalhousie funds were targeted for support of the Outpost Program. Funds at
McMaster, McGill and the University of British
Columbia were also considerable and it is probable
that in all three cases these were applied to both
graduate program development and research projects.
However, it is not possible to delineate the exact
purposes for which these funds were used in detail
as only the aggregate amounts were available.

By 1975-76 increases in the amounts of grants
were remarkable and more schools were reporting
research funds than had previously done so. With
one exception, all schools with graduate programs

reported receiving research monies that year. At the University of British Columbia, where the largest sum of funds received was reported ($489,629), the steadily rising percentage of university research funds being received by nursing is notable - from 0.27% in 1970-71 to 2.95% in 1975-76. Also at Toronto and McGill, which were both the recipients of much larger aggregate amounts of external grants in 1975-76, nursing's share of the university research enterprise in those large, complex, research-oriented institutions showed sharp increases. Toronto experienced a 51% increase in research funds over 1970-71 while McGill's increase was even larger at 79%. McMaster too had large external awards in 1975-76 which gave it an astounding 95% increase over the research funds it had received in 1970-71. Finally, two schools which had not received research funds in 1970-71 showed evidence of significant faculty development in the area of research expertise as both were awarded substantial research monies in 1975-76. Although Universite de Montreal had offered a graduate program since 1966, it might have been expected as the only French language graduate program in the country, to have become deeply involved in research. The University of Manitoba is quite another story, and an interesting one at that. In view of the development of faculty research resources at that university within a relatively short period of time, the receipt of $88,728 in research funds in the absence of a graduate program and despite the relatively short tenure of degree programs at that university is indeed remarkable. It should be noted that the figures reported for 1980-81 are based solely on the statistics in the *Reference List of Health Science Research in Canada* (1980), and thus there may well have been other grants to the schools of nursing in the various universities which have not been included in this list. There would not, however, appear to be substantially increased support for nursing research.

This review of the research funds received by university schools of nursing clearly indicates that developments in research have accompanied those in graduate education. With the increase in the number of faculty members qualified to staff graduate programs and the financial resources of schools offering programs, there has been a concomitant increase in the number of students seeking admission to the eight programs which are now operational. Concurrently there has been a considerable change in the nature and extent of the research enterprise stimulated by the sharply increased levels of federal funding for nursing research projects under the direction of nurse researchers who are faculty members in university schools of nursing.

REFERENCES

Bonneau, L.P., & Corry, J.A. (1972). *Quest for the optimum: Research policy in the universities of Canada.* Ottawa: Association of Universities and Colleges of Canada.

Defence Research Board. (1963). *Medical research projects completed in Canada, 1949-1963.* Ottawa: Author.

Defence Research Board. (1967). *Reference list of medical research projects in Canada.* Ottawa: Author.

Good, S.R. (1969). Submission to the study of of supportive research. In *Universities for the Science Secretariat of the Privy Council.* Ottawa: Canadian Nurses Association and Canadian Nurses Foundation.

Griffin, A. (1971). Nursing research in Canadian universities. In *National Conference on Research in Nursing Practice.* Ottawa: School of Nursing, University of British Columbia.

Harris, R.S. (1975). *A history of higher education in Canada: 1663-1960.* Toronto: The University of Toronto Press.

Imai, R. (1971). Associations and research activities. In *National Conference on Research and Nursing.* Ottawa: School of Nursing, University of British Columbia.

Medical Research Council. (1980). *Reference list of health science research in Canada.* Ottawa: Author.

National Conference of Canadian Universities (1944). *Proceedings.* Ottawa: Author.

Osmond, D.H. (1976). Sickness in Canada's health system. *The University of Toronto Graduate,* Spring.

Structure and Funding

Peitchinis, S.H. (1971). *Financing post secondary education in Canada*. Toronto: Council of Ministers of Education in Canada.

Poole, P.E. (1971). Research activities conducted or sponsored by government or service agencies. In *National Conference on Research in Nursing Practice*. Ottawa: School of Nursing, University of British Columbia.

Rowat, D.C. (1970). *The university, society in government: The report of the Commission on Relations between Universities and Governments*. Ottawa: University of Ottawa Press.

Secretary of State. (1975). *Review of educational policies in Canada: Government of Canada report*. Toronto: Council of Ministers of Education of Canada.

Spinks, J.W.T. (1962). Graduate studies and research in the sciences. In A.D. Duntan & D. Patterson (Eds.), *Canada's universities in a new age*. Ottawa: National Conference of Canadian Universities and Colleges.

Stinson, S.M. (1969). Deprofessionalization in nursing? Ed.D. dissertation. New York: Teachers College, Columbia University.

Stinson, S.M. (1977). Central issues in Canadian nursing research. In B. LaSor & M.R. Elliott (Eds.), *Issues in Canadian nursing*. Scarborough, Ontario: Prentice-Hall Canada Ltd.

Symons, T.H.B. (1975). *To know ourselves: The report of the Commission on Canadian Studies* (Vol. I & II). Ottawa: Association of Universities and Colleges of Canada.

Chapter Seven

IMPACT OF THE DIVISION OF NURSING ON RESEARCH DEVELOPMENT IN THE U.S.A.

Susan R. Gortner

HISTORICAL DEVELOPMENT OF THE DIVISION OF NURSING RESEARCH

The Federal interest in nursing research dates back to the period immediately following World War II, when nursing and other health leaders began to express growing concern about the quality and quantity of the nurse supply. Vreeland (1964), writing authoritatively on the first published history of the nursing research programs of the Public Health Service (PHS), refers to the number of requests for expert nurse consultation to both academic and service settings in order to resolve problems associated with nursing education and care delivery.

The requests apparently increased in urgency as a result of the implementation of the Cadet Nurse Corps program during World War II. That program prompted the collection of information by the United States Public Health Service (PHS) from practically all of the thirteen hundred schools of nursing then participating in the wartime effort. These national data provided state-by-state documentation of the extent and seriousness of some of the nursing education and nursing service problems facing the nation (Vreeland, 1964). The report, *Nursing Schools of the Mid Century*, prepared by PHS staff in collaboration with the National Committee for the Improvement of Nursing Service (West & Hawkins, 1950), gave momentum to the beginning of the accreditation program of the newly established (1952) National League for Nursing.

Since nurses were not returning to civilian service in the numbers anticipated after the war, the Federal leadership responded in 1948 by establishing the Division of Nursing Resources, and

Margaret Arnstein was appointed as chief of the new division. At the same time, Lucile Petry (Leone), who had administered the Cadet Nurse Corps program during the war, became the first Assistant Surgeon General of the Public Health Service and its Chief Nurse Officer. By attracting a small group of researchers, investigators, statisticians, social scientists, and consultants, these two individuals were instrumental in developing the intramural activities for which the Division came to be known. The Division of Nursing's historical files bear witness to the careful thinking, vision, and talent of this leadership in providing a small but important national nucleus of skilled personnel to guide the nursing research development effort. These staff members were responsible for devising and adapting methodologies for systematic study of nurse supply and distribution, job satisfaction and turnover, satisfaction with nursing care on the part of both personnel and patients, and documenting the quantity, quality, and cost of nursing education.

These activities produced a number of classic study manuals as an aid to state institutions and agencies to allow self-appraisal according to standards for statewide nursing services, appraisal of nursing service and outpatient departments, and the study of nursing activities in patient units (USDHEW, PHS, 1964; Stanford, 1957; Adams, 1957). Efforts of Division staff were directed to addressing and analysing these complex nursing and patient care problems. Some of the projects were of a program-oriented nature; others were individual investigations carried out by staff scientists.

The early Division staff are reported to have divided up the country into regions, visiting each frequently, and maintaining contacts and consulting with service and academic settings. An early commentary in *Nursing Research* suggests the level of energy and impact of the early consultant staff. Lucile Leone, Ellwynne Vreeland, Faye Abdellah, Helen Belcher, and Ava Dilworth interpreted the potentialities of research in nursing to universities and other research institutes, to nursing and medical schools, and to departments of biological and social sciences throughout the country during the first decade of Federal research activities. The importance of the contributions of members from other disciplines was recognised early and encouraged.

Early extramural work began just prior to 1950 with the award of several grants. Margaret

Arnstein of the Division of Nursing Resources and Elizabeth Stobo of the National Organisation for Public Health Nursing received funds from the PHS to develop a method for a cost analysis of public health nursing; later, supplements of this analysis were to assist public health agencies (Vreeland, 1958). During the same period of early extramural research awards, five other projects were funded, among them the important five-year curriculum research and evaluation project in basic nursing education of the University of Washington (Sand & Belcher, 1954), and the project conducted by Leo Simmons and associates at Yale University, which was a review of nursing studies and research over the past fifty years and done in collaboration with Virginia Henderson (Simmons & Henderson, 1964).

Priorities for Research Addressed
Interest in the nurse supply continued, and during the early 1950's, states began to study their needs and resources and to look at the factors influencing the preparation, progression, and retention of the pool of recruits into the nursing profession. Priorities for research were publicised by a number of nursing leaders. The Chief Nurse Officer (Lucile Petry Leone) wrote the first guest editorial for one of the early issues of the fledgling periodical *Nursing Research* (and prepared a special resume of the need for studies in research in nursing, in defense of the request to the Surgeon General in 1954 for extramural funds, program research grants and research fellowships). She encouraged the following areas of investigation: 1) recruitment, supply, education, and utilisation of nursing personnel for all types of nursing service; 2) identification of the relationships and responsibilities of nursing personnel; 3) development of methods for evaluating nursing care and education in all areas of nursing, both professional and non-professional; 4) ascertaining the relationship of nursing care to patient welfare; 5) exploration of the safety, comfort, and economy of various types of nursing units, equipment, and procedures used by nurses in caring for patients; 6) investigation of the interaction of nurses with others in multi-disciplinary patient care; 7) experimental studies of nursing methods and procedures in any field; and 8) studies of nursing as an occupation (Vreeland, 1958). In an internal memorandum to Leone, early in 1959, Vreeland went further to indicate the importance of the identification of

scientific content of nursing, and the seeking of and experimentation with new concepts of nursing; for example, the motivation or re-motivation of persons, and the careful study of the nursing care given by expert nurse practitioners to develop a body of descriptive information (as reported by Gortner & Nahm, 1977).

Establishment of the Grant and Fellowship Programs

These areas of proposed investigation illustrate one of the most important functions that the Division of Nursing and its antecedent, the Division of Nursing Resources, served for the entire nation. Because of the unique national position of Division scientific staff, and because of their continual contacts with the nursing academic and practice community, and with scientific activities in other fields, the staff were in an extraordinarily influential position to stimulate studies that would have an impact for decades to come. Long before the nursing literature began to address consistently the importance of scientific content for nursing, Vreeland and Leone were able to see the need for such inquiry, and to convince those in the Federal medical establishment, particularly the Surgeon General and the leadership of the National Institutes of Health, to allocate a portion of the Federal research budget to begin a program of extramural grants and fellowships for nursing. And so it was begun in 1955 with an initial allocation of $500,000 for the first year. A research branch and a fellowship branch were established in the Division of Nursing Resources, along the lines comparable to similar branches in the various institutes of the National Institutes of Health, with Vreeland as the first chief. In the fall of 1955, the first applications were received and reviewed (Vreeland, 1964; Gortner & Nahm, 1977). The importance of the structure and process for the early review of nursing research grant and fellowship applications cannot be underestimated. The structure was identical to that of other institutes in the various areas of medicine and biomedical science. The review process used the well-established mechanism of peer review, a two-stage review process in which initial review is done by a scientific study section, and is followed by further review for program development and policy considerations by a National Advisory Council (Vreeland, 1964; Gortner, 1971; Bloch, Gortner & Sturdivant, 1978).

NURSING RESEARCH SUPPORT

Initially, the grant awards were very modest, and ranged from several hundred to a few thousand dollars, and included a category of small grants and exploratory grants for pilot work. During the first few years, most of the awards were made to non-nurse investigators. After the early 60's, the picture began to change and by 1963, half of the principal investigators of the nursing projects were nurses (Vreeland, 1964). Other principal investigators on nursing research grants were medical scientists including physicians, educators, social and behavioral scientists, engineers, and hospital administrators. Currently four-fifths of investigators are nurses. It should be remembered that the Federal interest in health services research had not yet taken form in the Public Health Service reorganisation action of 1967, with the establishment of the National Center for Health Services Research. Thus, much of the early work that can now be called health services research was supported by nursing research grants. The first Public Health Service extramural awards for operations and systems research and appraisal of inpatient care services were supported with nursing research funds. In addition to the systems research projects, other projects investigated collaborative studies of medical and nursing practice with the same patients, in order to better differentiate professional roles and activities.

Vreeland's 1964 article reflects a beginning shift in priorities among the project grants supported, in which the relationship of nursing care to patient welfare is listed, first followed by development of methods for identifying patient needs and evaluating nursing care.

Attention is given to the various environments in which nursing care takes place and their influence on the quality and quantity of nursing.

RESEARCH TRAINING

Research resource development became an important programmatic activity of the newly formed research branch and fellowship branch, and was to take two major routes. The first was the use of the competitive fellowship mechanism to support promising individuals, in this instance, nurses for short term and long term research training. Again begun in 1955 and patterned after other NIH research training predoctoral fellowships, this program was intended to increase the numbers of scientists qualified to carry on independent research. Awards provided a modest stipend, as well as defrayment of tuition (and other academic fees). Additionally, part-time research fellowships were provided for those who could not undertake full-time work. These provided a cost per unit, plus indirect costs to schools of nursing to defray part-time study. Vreeland reported in 1958 that in the first three years of program effort, 78 full-time nursing research fellowships had been granted, and the number of awards for full-time study were increasing in proportion to the short-term awards, which at that point numbered 156. The short-term fellowship program ultimately was phased out in favor of long-term study as the needs for substantial grounding in research methods and basic and applied science became more apparent. Increasingly, the trends and applicants for the research fellowship program showed over the years a younger applicant pool, with broader academic and professional preparation, including a number of publications, and increasing studies in nursing as the discipline of choice in contrast to education. These trends were noted by Bourgeois (1975), and are further confirmed in terms of the present pool of fellows engaged in full-time study. An interesting recent development within the past five years has been the numbers of nurses undertaking postdoctoral work. Since 1956, twelve and one half million dollars have been spent to fund nearly two thousand awards to nurse research fellows enrolled in formal study.

Research resource development through research training took another form, again patterned after a successful mechanism of the National Institutes of Health, which was the Medical Scientist Training Program. Early in the 1960's it was apparent that individual fellowship support would be insufficient to accommodate nursing needs for trained scientific personnel. Accordingly, a Nurse Scientist Graduate Training Grant program was developed by Division staff with the major argument being that more nurses needed to receive preparation in the basic biological, physical, and social sciences related to nursing to increase the supply of competent nurse scientists while at the same time maintaining an identity in nursing. It will be remembered that a majority of the early fellowship awards were made to nurses seeking preparation in education, or administration. Some argued that the slow growth in practice related research was a function of the shortage of nurse investigators with preparation in the basic sciences.

The purpose of the Nurse Scientist Graduate Training Grants was to increase the numbers of nurses available for research and academic careers who were competent in the basic sciences, and who could contribute to the solution of health problems of the community, state, nation, and world by the application of knowledge in its most recent state of discovery. The grants were made on a competitive basis to qualified public and nonprofit institutions to establish, expand, and improve training opportunities in the health-related sciences for nurses interested in a career in research. In fiscal year 1962, two Nurse Scientist Graduate Training Grants were awarded, one to Boston University School of Nursing (for support of training in psychology, sociology, and biology), and the other to the University of California, San Francisco, School of Nursing, for study in sociology. In the next fiscal year, three additional Nurse Scientist Training Grants were awarded, one to the University of California, Los Angeles, School of Nursing, for graduate study in sociology; one to the University of Washington, School of Nursing, for graduate study in anthropology, microbiology, physiology, and sociology; and the third to Western Reserve University, School of Nursing, for study in biology, physiology, psychology, and sociology. Subsequently, the University of Kansas was awarded support for study in anatomy, physiology, psychology, sociology, and anthropology, as was Teachers College, Columbia University, for study in psychology. The University of Pittsburgh was granted support for study on maternal child health, and the Universities of Arizona and Colorado were granted support.

The competition for these grants and the application review process were vigorous. As was true then, and is true 20 years later, particular attention was given to the qualifications of the institution and its staff for teaching and research in the basic sciences important to research in nursing. Attention was paid to the research productivity and track record of the faculty members and the graduates of the training program in the relevant sciences. Other features of these institutional grants included opportunities for interdisciplinary study and research, and the availability of a well-qualified program director. The grants provide stipends to trainees selected by the institute, as well as to participating departments to help defray costs of instruction.

The institutional support for scientific training in nursing was based on early recognition of the relevance of the theories, laws, and principles within the basic sciences for professional fields such as nursing. It was felt important to have selected members of the profession obtain preparation in the basic sciences so that they in turn could identify and organise knowledge basic to nursing practice, and have the necessary preparation to address critical nursing questions through systematic inquiry. The nurse scientist produced by these programs became the university nurse faculty member of the next decade. The settings themselves were to be, in the main, the settings in which the Ph.D. programs in nursing were to develop (Cleland, 1979). The Nurse Scientist Graduate Training program, together with the original Individual Nurse Research Fellowship program, has provided the major means of support for the present investigator pool in the United States. The research training efforts have had a significant impact on the quality of nursing research and have enhanced both the graduate and undergraduate research training component in academic nursing settings nationwide. The Federal investments on behalf of research training have totalled $20,700,000 since 1955, of which $12,500,000 was for support of special fellowships, and the remainder for research training grants.[2]

DEVELOPMENT OF INSTITUTIONAL RESEARCH RESOURCES

As the nation's university-based nursing education programs began to develop their complement of resources and faculty more fully it became apparent that special emphasis would have to be given research activities and the establishment of research climates as well as resources all of which are important for the growth of graduate education. During the 1950's few nurse faculty members held earned doctorates, few could be released from their teaching responsibilities to conduct research, few could engage in formal study to upgrade their research skills, and a good portion of the nursing research ongoing at that time was being carried out by non-nurse investigators. Private and public funds were used from the late 1950's to the late 1960's to enable universities to conduct research seminars and provide formal and informal research assistance to their faculty. Also these funds were used to allow faculty released time from their teaching responsibilities, to provide supportive research services and purchase needed equipment, and to recruit research trained faculty. Public funds were administered through a special grant program known as the Faculty Research Development Grant. During the period 1958 through 1966, 21 such grants were awarded, 19 to schools conducting graduate programs, one to a school only conducting an undergraduate program, and one to a graduate school of public health. An evaluation of these grants revealed the following outcomes from the initial effort in institutional research development:

o recruitment and retention of research trained faculty;
o time and opportunity to participate in exploratory studies often dealing with patient care;
o the availability of consultation through the presence of a project director;
o the availability of supporting services;
o stimulation of ideas and creation of a favorable research climate; and
o establishment of a timetable or program for research which allowed the time and funds needed for the conduct of investigations (Schwartz, 1969).

For the next 15 years public and private funds continued to support the growth of institutional research resources. Noteworthy were a number of trends which changed the particular types of objectives and activities which comprised institutional development:

o considerable progress had been made during this time in increasing the number of nurses with earned doctorates;
o more nurses were able to obtain some research experience in their graduate programs through improved graduate education and improved means for student assistance;
o research had gained wider recognition as a requirement both of effective teaching and effective practice;
o climates within educational settings were more favorable towards research; and
o the health needs of the nation were becoming critical in the area of improved care and patient services.

Such private and public funds allowed the complementation and supplementation of research activities already initiated by the educational institution. In contrast to the earlier efforts, less emphasis was given to the upgrading or training of faculty in elementary methods of research and more emphasis was given to the conduct of actual investigations and to discussions of persistent problems both of a substantive and methodological nature. Batey (1978) carried out a review of 12 settings that had had research development funds noting the factors associated with research productivity.

Because institutional research resources are necessary for a wide complement of research and teaching activities, it was often difficult to justify both their need as well as their impact. Non-categorical, i.e. nonspecific, funds for support of research, such as those of the Division's Research Development Grant Program and the Biomedical Research Support Grant Program of the NIH (Gortner, 1973), did support a variety of much-needed activities essential both to basic and graduate education, to the advancement of knowledge, and to the application of research findings to the field. Increasingly, schools of nursing were able to draw on intramural (university) as well as private funds for support of a variety of institutional activities.

In 1978 and 1979 two categorical programs of research support were announced by the Division of Nursing. Nursing research program grants were established in 1978 to stimulate the conduct of clusters of studies focused upon a single theme, in order to substantially enlarge the body of scientific knowledge basic to nursing practice, education, and administration. It was expected that, in this manner, nursing research efforts might become more focused than is presently the case, and that institutions would be able to enlarge their nursing research programs, resources, and outputs. Program grants encompassed three or more studies which 'may investigate common questions in different populations, or explore different aspects of the single theme in varying ways, but every study in the group would have as its research goal the investigation of some dimension of the single theme....' Principal investigators of such program grants were to be experienced nurse researchers, with each component project headed by a different project director in order to stimulate cooperative research and permit different perspectives to the research.

The announcement of the availability of nursing research program grants was received with a great deal of enthusiasm by the nursing research community. Division of Nursing staff soon found that the development of an application consisting of a group of co-ordinated studies was not an easy task for researchers, many of whom had never before submitted an individual research proposal to rigorous national scientific scrutiny. It has been suggested that novice researchers cooperate as a group in a single research grant application, prior to launching a multiproject venture. Six program grants have been funded by the Division of Nursing since the inception of the program, and their life is too short to assess adequately their impact.

Another variant of Division of Nursing programs to strengthen the research capabilities of schools of nursing is the program of Nursing Research Emphasis Grants for Doctoral Programs in Nursing (NRE/DPN), which was announced as an one-time effort in 1979.

In the 1970's, schools of nursing developed doctoral programs at a significantly increasing pace, creating concern on the part of many nurse educators about the adequacy of the research base upon which some of the doctoral programs were developed. In this vein, the prestigious Committee on a Study of National Needs for Biomedical and Behavioral Research Personnel of the National Academy of Sciences, in its 1978 report, expressed its concern that the research strength of schools of nursing with doctoral programs is quite variable (Committee, 1978).

The Division of Nursing decided, therefore, to specifically design a grant program to assist schools of nursing with doctoral programs to enhance their research base.

The major purpose of the program was to strengthen the research efforts and resources of faculty members, and to stimulate the development of nursing research (basic and applied) in specific areas of emphasis relating to the health of vulnerable families and groups.[4] Suggested were the following areas: 1) children; for example, studies concerned with stress of hospitalisation or studies dealing with terminal illness; 2) adolescents; for example, studies relating to adolescent pregnancy or parenting skills; 3) beginning families and parenting; including studies concerned with care in innovative settings, such as birth centers, or problems of parent-child relationships; 4) aged, chronically ill, or terminally ill; including studies concerned

with alternatives to hospitalisation, and enhance-
ment of the quality of life; and 5) minorities and
underserved groups; including studies of their
unique health problems, and studies concerned with
access and barriers to care.

The inclusion in the application of plans for
specific studies to be carried out with this grant
support was mandatory, but it was expected that
such studies would be small, exploratory, and to be
supported for a relatively brief period. The
expectation was that this support would stimulate
faculty to begin to lay the groundwork necessary
prior to the submission of an independent grant
application. Participation of doctoral students as
research assistants in faculty research projects
was strongly encouraged.

That the program was received with immense
enthusiasm is evidenced by the fact that 22 out of
23 eligible schools made an application. Many
applicants subsequently reported that the development of the application in and of itself was a
beneficial experience because it stimulated faculty
members interested in research to come together, to
do a self-assessment, and to cooperate in the
making of plans and in the development of an application. These applications were subjected to the
usual review, and 13 have been funded. Recent
analysis of the projects indicates that three
schools are generally concentrating on beginning
families and parenting, two schools on the aged,
three schools on the chronically ill, and one on
the concept 'social support', while four address
multiple content areas.

Again, it is too early to evaluate the impact
of these projects, but it would appear the combined
research and doctoral program features have benefited faculty research efforts and doctoral student
training.

**RESEARCH ON THE DEVELOPMENT OF A SCIENTIFIC BASE
FOR PRACTICE**

The late 1960's began an important reorientation of
the Federal interest in nursing research with
particular attention being given to studies that
would be relevant to patient care issues and problems. Following the establishment of the National
Center for Health Services Research, in 1967, some
nursing research grant project investigators moved
their research efforts into the field of health
services research in general. Thus the Division of

Nursing research branch staff devoted its attention, with the help of its scientific advisory committee (then called the Nursing Research and Patient Care Review Committee), to a review of accomplishments in the first 15 years of the program, and to the areas of research that would need to be addressed in the submission of research grant applications.

A decided effort again was made to stimulate the nature and development of nursing research studies, regionally, with branch staff visiting the colleges and universities and service settings, attending regional and national meetings, and providing consultation directly to potential applicants. This tremendous effort on the part of the staff, as well as the study section consultants, resulted in an increase of applications, both in number and quality, after 1971.

In a relatively brief time, the number of applications dealing with clinical investigations directly related to aspects of nursing practice doubled. Because of this increase, an attempt was made by Division of Nursing research branch staff to categorise the research into a number of major content areas: 1) the science of practice; 2) the artistry of practice; 3) the structures needed for optimal delivery of patient care; and 4) the tools or methods needed for assessment of practice. Systematic identification of various characteristics, health problems, and health needs of persons and groups of persons were the major thrust of the first category; the laboratory and field studies that evaluated the efficacy of nursing procedures, techniques, and methods were the focus of the second category. Descriptive, analytical, and experimental studies that examined the physical and social environments in which nurses and clients interact as well as patterns of health care delivery were subsumed under the third. Studies that aimed to develop methods for assessing patient welfare and care and that undertook to construct instruments appropriate to nursing research were in the fourth category, and the final dealt with the application of research findings (Gortner, Bloch & Phillips, 1976).

These categories have been found useful by such organisations as the American Association of Colleges of Nursing, by other authors documenting the evolution of nursing research in the United States, and by the Division of Nursing which used the categories to classify research grants on an annual basis until 1979. The number of studies with a clinical focus and addressing fundamental or applied scientific questions has been steadily increasing over the past decade. There has been a companion effect in methodology, with several important tools and compilation of tools arising both from grant-supported work and contracted work undertaken by the Division of Nursing. Over a 27 year period 65 million dollars has been invested in nursing research grants and contracts by the Division of Nursing.[5] It has served as the most prevalent source of funding for research in nursing, and for those studies brought to the publication stage.

SCIENTIFIC COMMUNICATION: RESEARCH CONFERENCE

The impact of the Division of Nursing on research development in the United States would not be complete without a brief description of the importance of Division support and use of the conference mechanism. Beginning in the late 1950's and continuing for the next 20 years, grants were made to individuals to bring together investigators in various parts of the country to address first problems of interest in clinical research and then to begin the network of scientific communication that has characterized other professional associations. Perhaps the greatest impact was felt through the conduct of the annual research conferences sponsored by the American Nurses Association between 1964 and 1973 that were supported through Federal grants. These conferences provided the first experience for nurse investigators to present papers, to have them critiqued, and to grow in the art of sophistication of scientific communication. Some have attributed the formation of the Council of Nurse Researchers, the first such membership group in the American Nurses Association, to the scientific communication network developed under these annual conferences with Federal support. The purposes of the first conferences were to provide opportunities for nurses engaged in research to examine critically and discuss selected research reports. The last conferences addressed various topics and used the format of simultaneous sessions and formal critiques. Over nine annual conferences the quality of research reported demonstrated a growth in understanding of comprehensive designs and increasing skill in critical analysis of research on the part of the participants. Similarly a series of six annual research meetings under the sponsorship of the Western Council for Higher

Education in Nursing between 1968 and 1973 was supported with Division of Nursing funds. The purposes of these regional conferences were similar to the national ANA conferences and prompted the formation of the Western Society for Research in Nursing which has continued the annual conference mechanism following termination of Federal support.

In addition to these general conference features, a number of special conferences around topics such as quality of care assessment, were supported through grant funds. The Division of Nursing Research Branch undertook the sponsorship of a number of invitational conferences on such topics as future directions for doctoral preparation in nursing, the nature of the nurse scientist graduate training program and the national needs for doctorally prepared manpower, assessment of nursing services and quality of care, and most recently an invitational conference to address future directions in knowledge for practice. This last conference provided an capstone for nearly a generation of Division of Nursing support of research development efforts in the United States, and brought together a number of distinguished individuals to look at the mechanisms for advancing nursing research, to address the areas of importance in nursing practice, and to examine the theoretical and scientific bases for practice. The major papers for that conference were published in the July-August 1980 issue of *Nursing Research*, together with a conference summary by Heinrich and Bloch (1980).

SUMMARY

This documentary of the impact of the Division of Nursing's research efforts on research development in the United States has necessarily been selective. It has concentrated on the activities and influence of the nursing research branch through the mechanisms of staff consultation and leadership, grants to individuals and institutions, fellowship and training grant support, and use of the contract and conference mechanism. It is difficult to imagine that nursing research would have flourished or grown so rapidly in its development had not this important resource been available to investigators and universities for assistance, and if a decision had not been made early on to use a portion of the public tax dollar in support of nursing research and research training activities.

For this early vision, the investigators in the United States are indebted. It is hoped that in the latter part of this century, the subject matter of nursing research can increasingly attract national attention and support.

NOTES

Acknowledgement: The assistance of Dr. Doris Bloch, Chief of the Research Support Section, Nursing Research Branch, Division of Nursing, in the review of an early draft of this manuscript and in providing fiscal data and information on program and emphasis grants is gratefully acknowledged.

1. Division of Nursing, Nursing Research Branch, 1981 Fiscal Summary Data. Unpublished.

2. Division of Nursing, Nursing Research Branch, 1981 Fiscal Summary Data. Unpublished.

3. Announcement of the Nursing Research Emphasis/Doctoral Program Grant, Division of Nursing, 1978.

4. Announcement of the Nursing Research Emphasis/Doctoral Program Grant, Division of Nursing, 1979.

5. Division of Nursing, Nursing Research Branch, 1981 Fiscal Summary Data. Unpublished.

REFERENCES

Adams, A.O. (1964). *How to study the nursing service of an outpatient department* (DHEW, U.S. Public Health Service Publication No. 497). Washington, DC: U.S. Government Printing Office.

Batey, M. (1978). *Research development in university schools of nursing.* Bureau of Health Manpower (DHEW Publication No. HRA 78-67). Hyattsville MD: U.S. Department of Health, Education and Welfare.

Bloch, D., Gortner, S.R., & Sturdivant, L.W. (1978). The nursing research grants program of the Division of Nursing, United States Public

Health Service. *Journal of Nursing Administration, 7,* 40-45.

Bourgeois, M.J. (1975). The special nurse research fellow: Characteristics and recent trends. *Nursing Research, 24,* 184-188.

Cleland, V.S. (1979). Educational issues related to research in nursing. In F.S. Downs & J.W. Fleming (Eds.), *Issues in nursing research.* New York: Appleton-Century-Crofts.

Commission on Human Resources (1978). Personnel needs and training for biomedical and behavioral research. The 1978 report of the *Committee on a Study of National Needs for Biomedical and Behavioral Research Personnel.* Washington, DC: National Academy of Sciences.

Gortner, S.R. (1973). The federal interest and grant programs. *American Journal of Nursing, 73,* 1052-1055.

Gortner, S.R., & Nahm, H. (1977). An overview of nursing research in the United States: I. Historical perspectives; II. Research developments in nursing education; III. The development of research in nursing practice; IV. The development of research resources. *Nursing Research, 26,* 10-33.

Gortner, S.R., Bloch, D., & Phillips, T. (1976). Contributions of nursing research to patient care. *Journal of Nursing Administration, 6,* 22-28.

Heinrich, J.R., & Bloch, D. (1980). Summary of "knowledge for practice" conference group discussions. *Nursing Research, 29,* 218.

Sand, O., & Belcher, H. (1954). Curriculum research in basic nursing education: A progress report. *Nursing Outlook, 2,* 86-89.

Schwartz, D. (1969). *Follow-up assessment of 19 FaRaDeg programs* (Final Report, Cornell University USPHS Nursing Research Grant NU-00307). Division of Nursing, U.S. Public Health Service.

Simmons, L.W., & Henderson, V. (1964). *Nursing research: A survey and assessment.* New York: Appleton-Century-Crofts.

Stanford, E.D. (1957). *How to study supervisor activities in a hospital nursing service.* (DHEW, Public Health Service Publication No. 496). Washington, DC: U.S. Government Printing Office.

United States Department of Health, Education and Welfare (1964). *How to study nursing activities in a patient unit.* (Public Health Service Publication No. 370). Washington, DC: U.S. Government Printing Office. (Revised)

Vreeland, E. (1958). The nursing research grant and fellowship program of the Public Health Service. *American Journal of Nursing, 58,* 1700-1702.

Vreeland, E. (1964). Nursing research programs of the Public Health Service. *Nursing Research, 13,* 148-158.

West, M., & Hawkins, C. (1950). *Nursing schools at the mid-century.* New York: National Commission for the Improvement of Nursing Services (p. 88).

PART III: PREPARATION FOR NURSING RESEARCH

Chapter Eight

NURSING RESEARCH AND NURSING PRACTICE: IMPLICATIONS
FOR UNDERGRADUATE RESEARCH

Marian McGee

NURSING RESEARCH DEVELOPMENT: UNDERGRADUATE

The ability to make the transition from the everyday world of nursing practice to the more remote
and unfamiliar realm of nursing research becomes a
career requisite for the ongoing acquisition of
knowledge essential for continuing professional
competence. Since the role of research consumer is
an important sphere of the staff nurse's *modus
operandi,* there is a need to provide an introduction to research at the undergraduate level. The
purpose of this chapter is to establish the relationship between nursing research and nursing
practice, the theme being that research skill is,
in a sense, an extension of clinical skill. As
nursing is a practice discipline, mastery of nursing research requires familiarity with the process
and content of nursing practice. This writer
believes that the assumption underlying this linkage is critical to the development of nursing
science and professional attitudes in students. In
this chapter, the author presents a comparison of
the research and problem solving processes and
considers attributes of the research process which
are believed to merit attention.

Research and Problem Solving
The problem solving process and the research process have much in common. Since students of nursing utilise problem solving in the form of nursing
process, the research process can be viewed as an
extension of an activity which is already understood. The basic assumption that precedes the
problem solving process differs only somewhat from
that which is antecedent to the research process.

In problem solving, one assumes there is an impediment to desired or normal performance. In the research process one assumes there is a factor which is of unknown relationship to the focus of attention; that is there is an irritant or an impediment to understanding or objective achievement.

When a clinical problem is identified, such identification is based on relevant data. Once the problem is identified, problem resolution becomes the goal with intermediate objectives as milestones to that achievement. For example, a patient with a fractured femur is immobilized. To restore and retain mobility is the health care objective. To achieve that objective, it is the role of medicine to assure alignment and await calcification. Nursing has a slightly more complex task in that skin integrity, cast or crutch walking, rest, exercise and feelings of security, and coping must be promoted and protected. Experience in solving particular problems allows the practitioner to predict outcomes with some degree of certainty. This only holds, of course, if associated factors and circumstances are essentially similar from situation to situation. Practitioners find it difficult to handle items or factors whose relationship with the problem is either unclear or varies with the situation. As a consequence, it becomes essential to identify if those factors that seem to be associated with the problem are attributes of the problem or perhaps related to the cause or outcome.

One of the reasons for classification is to handle variance and to organise characteristics according to the degree of variance. It is much easier to handle five groups with relatively similar characteristics than to plan care for twenty-five people viewing each in single isolation. To derive meaning from the classification, or in other words manipulate the data statistically, one requires a minimal number in each group. I would suggest that no clinician assumes an individual to be truly unique.

Thus, it is necessary that we have a process of investigation providing order and sequence in the study. The first step in any investigation, whether it is in practice or in research, is to determine the problem. Most questions or most problems initially identified by investigators are much too broad or vague. There are too many variables and impinging factors to be managed. The question must be narrowed down or the problem must

be clearly delineated. The next step is to identify the objectives. The objective becomes an even
more explicit focus of attention than was the
problem. Each problem usually involves several
objectives; the selection of the research objective
is a selection of one from among many. Concomitant
with the identification of the research objective
must go the identification of the assumptions
associated with that objective. This particular
determination is probably one of the most difficult
steps in the research process. Browne and
Pallister (1981) graphically demonstrated the
proportion of total effort that must be allocated
to problem identification and formulation of hypothesis.

It is difficult to identify all of the factors
which may be related to any one problem. For
example, in the past we have assumed that patients
with fractures were victims of some impacting force
or a fall. Consequently, investigators and practitioners searched for hazardous structures in the
environment or dizziness and imbalance in victims.
Recent work in geriatrics has revealed that frequently spontaneous fractures may precede a fall in
the elderly. This suggests that the fracture
results in falling as opposed to a fracture being
the result of a fall.

A tabulation is presented as a vehicle for
comparison of the two processes and a demonstration
of their similarity (see Table 8.1).

A difference between the two processes can be
found in the probability of replication. In problem solving, the extent to which the process can be
repeated with the same outcome is frequently unknown (other than intuitively or experientially).
In the research process, the probability of replication is known and documented. Another difference
is in the generalisability of the results. Because
there is greater control through sampling and
standardised procedure, it can be predicted that
the results will hold true in the larger population
or larger context, for example, 90 percent of the
time or 70 percent of the time. To contrast research and problem solving we can use elements
identified by Popham (1975) to contrast research
and evaluation (see Table 8.2).

In summary, research is the systematic investigation of any phenomenon. It is an extension of
problem solving. The extension is related to
repeatable data control. Because one wishes to be
able to repeat the process and have the same outcome each time, *prediction* becomes a critical

TABLE 8.1

COMPARISON OF THE PROBLEM SOLVING PROCESS
AND THE RESEARCH PROCESS

STEP	PROBLEM SOLVING PROCESS	RESEARCH PROCESS
One	Identify the obstacle - take a history or screen and diagnose	Identify the irritant (the research problem) Determine the frequency (if possible) of its manifestation and describe its context
Two	Confirm the objective - identify desired outcomes to nursing action(s)	Confirm what you wish to learn (i.e., the research objective)
Three	Identify alternative routes to the objective	Specify the variable relationship i.e., the relationship between intervention and outcome, or cause and effect, or direction and association (in a population)

TABLE 8.1 (continued)

STEP	PROBLEM SOLVING PROCESS	RESEARCH PROCESS
Four	Identify the necessary resources, costs or effort, benefits or pay-off, mechanisms	Design the mode of inquiry (how to observe) Determine the sampling requirements Select or formulate the instruments Develop a coding system Identify content and sequence of observation
Five	Sequence the subtasks of each alternative	Organize resources in relation to action plan
Six	Determine feasibility	Collect, code, keypunch data Select statistic(s)
Seven	Determine clinical significance Choose most desirable alternative	Analyse, compare and contrast data groups Determine degree of difference between groups Determine statistical significance
Eight	Implement	Draw conclusions
Nine	Evaluate, i.e., was objective achieved?	Interpret

TABLE 8.2

A CONTRAST OF RESEARCH AND PROBLEM SOLVING

Characteristic*	Research*	Problem Solving
1. Focus of inquiry	conclusion understanding	impediment removal
2. Generalizability of results	high	low
3. Role of valuing in inquiry	unimportant sufficient to discover truth	important
4. Measurement principles	essential	less important
5. Scientific principles	essential	useful
6. Description	sufficient, or not necessary	not necessary not sufficient
7. Judgement	not necessary not sufficient	necessary sufficient
8. Sampling techniques	crucial	not necessary

TABLE 8.2 (continued)

Characteristic*	Research*	Problem Solving
9. Random selection of subjects	important if possible	not important
10. Descriptive and Inferential Statistics	utilized	may be utilized
11. Audience	may or may not be identified	identified and important
12. Politics	improper	recognized
13. Replicability	important	usually not possible
14. Setting	may or may not be important	important
15. Reporting	external	internal
16. Theory building	important	unimportant

* Popham, 1975

purpose of research. Because one wishes to learn the cause of a problem, *identification* becomes a critical purpose and because one wishes to understand the problem, *explanation* becomes a critical purpose. Research is meant to identify, explain and predict those factors, concerns and issues with a greater certainty than would otherwise be possible.

Problem Identification and Nursing Research

Talking about problem delineation is easier than accomplishing it in fact. The knowledge about that which has piqued one's curiosity has a direct relationship to the ease with which the problem can be delineated. For example, are particular strategies of counselling or of health education more efficacious than others in preventing family dysfunction or improving family function?

In these irritants, there are several assumptions and, potentially, several research objectives. There are assumptions about the constituents or ingredients of family function as well as the validity of indicators of those ingredients. Many families receive considerable attention and nursing care without appreciable evidence of change in health practices and coping. Does the problem lie with the family? Its particular structure and functional style? The circumstances of the family? The strategies of nursing intervention? Or the laws of chance? If health practices have both cognitive and affective dimensions, and if families function as a unit, then do families, as a unit, have an identifiable learning style? There must be an identifiable profile that characterizes the group to earn the label of family as a unit. It follows that the items which serve as indicators must be observable and quantifiable as well as being true indicators of the phenomenon.

The implication is that an investigator must invest considerable thought before even addressing the relevant literature. One must also convince oneself of the relationship of the question to nursing. One's conceptual framework for nursing practice is the framework with which the clinical research problem must articulate. It might be necessary to address the literature the first time at this point, unless this conceptual homework is already completed. If so, the gap or discrepancy in clinical practice related to, for example, learning styles, the content of health behaviour, family theories and nursing strategies, can be closed by pursuing the literature to determine why the problem is perceived as such. To solve clinical problems or identify researchable problems, one must be sensitive to the probability of the existence of the problem. The frequency with which the problem or condition is manifested in a practice, or in a population, supplies the necessary impetus for investigatory pursuit and for problem resolution.

The relevant literature, one's own experience and the experience of the discipline must come together. As in clinical practice, one is constantly challenged to identify the obstacles to objectives, acquire the information needed to devise and select the strategies that have some probability of success in obstacle control or removal.

Problem Distribution
The notions of probability theory obtain throughout in both the process of investigation and in nursing practice. Part of the problem definition in research is its distribution in a population and that distribution is expressed in the form of observed frequency or expected frequency. Any time anyone is operating in terms of the expected, one is applying probability with greater or lesser reliability. In research, one invests considerable effort in controlling bias, chance and artifact in order to strengthen the statements of probability of frequency. In clinical problem solving, one most frequently does not have time to build in those controls, i.e. to wait for an answer that has been confirmed through unbiased testing or observation. Nevertheless, the clinical decision-making is carried out on the basis of belief in the frequency with which: a problem is seen; a strategy works; or a symptom (i.e. indicator) reflects a clinical problem.

Inference
Nursing history forms are developed because of the reliance (intuitive or otherwise) on applied probability. Each item on a history form must have particular utility in determining the probability of problem existence (or in determining the necessity to depart from the standard care plan). The history tool screens for that decision. By the same token, the investigator uses a questionnaire

or observation schedule, or an adequate sample, to determine the extent to which the subjects conform to criteria or vary in terms of the items in the instrument. Inference about the relationship of variables (items) in terms of the study population can be drawn only after the quantified data have been subjected to statistical tests. Whereas the clinician uses previously reported research or an educated guess to support inference, an investigator attempts to supply evidence for inference.

Significance
The concept of significance is equally critical to the practitioner and the investigator and for the same reasons. There is a difference, however. It is suggested that significance has two dimensions. One dimension addresses the relationship of the variable to the clinical problem and the client, and so the presenting picture has *clinical significance*. Many decisions are made in clinical practice which are based on clinically significant indicators. A pulse rate of 80 under certain circumstances is clinically significant.

The other dimension of significance relates to quantification and the degree to which the observation or indicator is manifested in a population or between groups. Such significance is *statistical* and is a result that reflects a confirmed difference between a control group and an experimental group or between actual and expected outcomes. Statistical significance only means that the probability of the observed phenomenon being one of chance is limited, e.g. to one in a hundred (0.01) or perhaps one in a thousand (0.001). It is suggested also that the statistical criterion the investigator chooses should be a function of the clinical significance of the measure.

Error
As one wishes to control error in clinical decision-making, so one wishes to do this in research decisions. The probability of error is the main target for control in both the clinical and the research processes. One constantly attempts to diminish error that is a function of the investigator bias (invalid assumptions, unreliable data) or is a function of systematic bias (inadequate or improper sampling). For an introduction to data control and statistical manipulation, the student is referred to a text entitled *Statistical Literacy: A Guide to*

Interpretation (Haack, 1979). The notions of error, variance and deviation are smoothly handled in this readable non-threatening publication. There is a decision point however, where the clinician and the investigator must choose between two errors. The risk of these errors are experienced by all disciplines. By some, they are referred to as Type I and Type II errors (the most common reference); by some, they are called alpha and beta errors; and in health science practice they are associated with measures of sensitivity and specificity. A *Type I error* occurs when one rejects a valid or true hypothesis (or concludes a person is not ill when in fact he is sick). A *Type II error* occurs when the decision-maker fails to reject a false hypothesis (i.e. assumes someone is ill or has hypertension when in fact he does not). In clinical practice, we have been trained to elect the Type II error.

Earlier, we discussed the decisions of screening and suggested the screening mission is to identify those persons who are at high risk of experiencing a problem or who, we believe, are actually experiencing a problem. We use measures or indicators that will be sensitive (i.e. the patient would fail the test and the results would be labelled positive). The mission of screening is to include everyone who has or might have the problem. A Type II error is deliberately chosen in preference to the Type I and the indicators or tests have a *measure of sensitivity*. The resulting group will contain all persons who are test positive, but only some of whom actually have the problem. Those who do not have the problem were false positive.

The clinician then proceeds to do a diagnostic workup. In this aspect, he or she wishes to continue to avoid a Type I error. The decision-making is to rule out competing hypothesis or differentiating diagnoses. Here one requires specificity of "diagnostic" tests. For example, a glucose tolerance test is "diagnostic" for diabetes, whereas a fasting blood sugar is a screening test. The first has a *measure of specificity* and the second a *measure of sensitivity*. The test results of both will contain false positives and true positives, false negatives and true negatives. In screening, we wish to have as few false positives as possible.

Levels of Nursing Research and the Models of Research

The classification of research models is helpful to understand the role research plays in the development of our science, the confirmation of our practice and the boundaries of nursing function. Diers (1974) has clearly explicated the four levels of investigation initially articulated by James and Dickoff (1968).

The first level is *factor isolating* or investigation for the purpose of factor identification. Descriptive studies would fall under this rubric. The intent is to identify and delineate the relevant characteristics (or variables) in a situation or syndrome (problem, condition). This is a most fundamental level of research and most frequently the data are nominal. Attributes such as sex, address, eye colour are nominal data, which means the item is being used as a descriptor. For example, unless graduating shades of blue eyes is the focus of research measurement, eye colours (blue, green, brown) are assumed to be mutually exclusive. Place of residence is another item that is not usually measured, but rather is used as a descriptor. As a consequence, data items or attributes that cannot be measured are referred to as nominal-data. To identify the attributes associated with a problem or phenomenon is the investigator's first imperative and so factor-isolating research is the first level of nursing research. There are examples of this level elsewhere in this text, but Johnson and Hardin described the function of public health nursing in a classic descriptive study in 1962 (Johnson & Hardin, 1962).

Factor relating investigations address the indication of association. That is the determination of whether two or more characteristics or variables are manifested in some way together. For example, are people with red hair also likely to have blue eyes? Is the incidence of completed nursing care plans positively associated with reports by patients of feeling safe and well cared for? The factors are not seen as causally related, merely that where one is, the other is also found. That is, if A then also B.

Diers refers to this kind of study as "relation-searching". She suggests that other names for the study type are exploratory or descriptive. The line between the factor-isolating investigations and factor-relating investigations seems blurred at times. In the latter however, the factors or variables have already been identified as attributes of the phenomenon under study, but their relationship is not clear. Jones, in her work on nursing diagnosis, has put considerable effort into determining the factors relating to labels assigned by nurses to patient problems (Jones, 1979). The data in factor-relating studies are usually nominal as in factor-isolating but may achieve ordinality. For example, fatigue can be classified under mild, moderate and severe. Severe is more than moderate which is more than mild, but how much more is unclear.

Situation-relating or situation-predicting is the third level of investigation. The investigator is attempting to do more than discover the frequency with which a relationship is manifested; she is attempting to predict the level of an association. Epidemiological studies of relative risk in such associations as smoking and lung cancer are classic examples of this level of investigation. Very few nursing studies can as yet be assigned this rank.

A possible explanation for this lag in the development of nursing science is in the arduous, painful evolution of theories of, and for, nursing practice. Until the discipline has a critical mass of nursing researchers in pursuit of the articulation and validation of the elements of nursing in terms of nursing process, or clinical problem solving, nursing research will continue to languish at the descriptive level. The ability to render clinical judgement is founded on empirically-based prediction. Correlational, quasi-experimental and experimental designs are necessary to this task. The data must be at least interval data. That is, the calibration must be explicit and known.

Situation-producing is the most advanced level of investigation but not necessarily the most complex in design. In this level, prescriptions for desired outcomes are being tested. It is herein suggested that some designs of evaluative research achieve this status. Programmes or strategies are designed and implemented to resolve some clinical problem or control some risk factor. The subsequent (or concurrent) *controlled* investigation to determine the efficacy of the strategy is evaluative research. Clinical drug trials are examples of prescription testing or situation-producing studies. It might be worthy to note that only applied disciplines are likely to engage in this type of investigation.

The classic studies of Sackett, et al., are good examples of investigations which can be ranked as situation-producing or evaluative research. In a series of studies based at the McMaster University and using a consumer/provider population in Burlington, Ontario, Sackett and his colleagues demonstrated the efficacy of utilising nurse practitioners in health care delivery (Sackett et al, 1974).

Situation-producing research must utilise interval data, at least, and ratio data are preferable. Measures of light, heat and space provide ratio data. In these measures, the zero point is known and is identifiable. As a consequence, additions and multiplications can be specified. The zero point of economic resource is challenging, even to the imagination.

Research literacy is requisite to mastery of the process, and the foregoing section reflects the relationships of the role of research to both clinical practice and the development of nursing science. Literacy assumes a comprehension of the process, utilisation of criteria for validity and an appreciation of the relationship of these dimensions to nursing science and practice.

A Perspective for Learning/Teaching Nursing Research

The following grid is presented as an overview of the relationship of research type in terms of the four levels by year of program, the learning thrust for that year in terms of research related or support content and the level objective for the year. It would seem that in the first year of any nursing program one is being introduced to those subjects and content that relate most closely to nursing such as the social sciences, the biological sciences, communication and the ensocialization of nursing. By that, is meant that students are being introduced to what will be their main profile of clients, the process and behaviour of interaction and the mission of nursing. It follows then that a student is being encouraged to learn how to identify relevant data, to describe situations and to study man, man as a patient, man as a class of consumers. The learning thrust that relates both to beginning introduction to investigation also relates to beginning introduction to patient care. They learn to describe first the situation, to organise their data, to determine what these descriptors are, when a descriptor is relevant and when it is not. The level of judgment required here in order to determine the relevance of data being collected is of considerable interest for

TABLE 8.3

LEARNING/TEACHING NURSING RESEARCH

by Year and Focus

LEVEL AND TYPE OF RESEARCH	LEARNING THRUST	RELATED CONTENT	OBJECTIVE
YEAR I Factor isolating - descriptive - case study	Situation description - data organization - nominal grouping - concept of exclusivity - data collection - observation - interview	- sociology - physiology - nursing I - communication - psychology	- to understand data grouping & control
YEAR II Factor relating - exploratory - survey	- problem definition - problem identification - concept of association - datum relevance - measurement ordinality frequencies	- nursing process - developmental psychology - decision theory - nursing theories - nursing diagnosis	- to use inference - collate data

TABLE 8.3 (continued)

LEVEL AND TYPE OF RESEARCH	LEARNING THRUST	RELATED CONTENT	OBJECTIVE
YEAR III Situation-predicting - correlational analysis - quasi-experimental design	- measures of relative risk, central tendency - development & use of interval and ratio data - dependent & independent variable relationship - concept & criteria for: causality, reliability, correlation, sensitivity, specificity	- nursing process - nursing theories - nursing diagnosis	- to understand designs of investigation - use terminology of controlled investigation - identify research objective - generate hypothesis

YEAR IV Situation-prescribing
- evaluation
- cohort analysis
- clinical trials
- experimental
	- indicators & measure of intervention efficacy
	- critical analysis
	- models of research
	- linkage of nursing care & nursing problem to quantified indications of:
	  - adequacy
	  - appropriateness
	  - effectiveness
	  - efficiency
		nursing theories
		epidemiology
		theories of evaluation
			research literacy
			propose an investigation
			critique a research project

both education and practice. We practice collecting the data, observing the patient and eliciting information as well as communicating with patients or subjects. The objective is to understand the grouping of data and the control of the data. That is, what data should be included and what data should be excluded in the description.

Year two in a program moves more closely toward practice in the nursing process and in identifying problems. Problem definition becomes the focus of teaching and learning and it follows that the extent and mode of interpreting the various factors associated with the problem receive the most attention. The objective is to use inference, to collate the collected data, to be able to make a judgement so that the concept of association, data relevance, the notion of measurements with ordinality in frequency distributions become an important areas of skill development as well as of conceptual understanding. The associated type of research is exploratory or survey. Related content is nursing process. Developmental psychology is taught after the introduction to the field is accomplished. It assumes the student is ready to appreciate how the organism evolves to maturity, as well as what is believed and what is known about that evolution. Decision theory, nursing theories and nursing diagnostic process as well as related content are critical. The second level (or year) requires the attainment of knowledge and skill in these areas before pursuing the ability to predict both for research purposes as well as for the purpose of clinical decision-making.

Year three provides a learner with the opportunity to learn to predict situations. It is more complex both in an actual completion as well as in preparation for it. By this time, a student has developed some skill in applying the principles of the nursing process. Nursing theories are part of our armamentarium and the more complex dimensions of pathophysiology, pharmacology and biostatistics offer additional vehicles enhancing the ability to detect, the ability to segregate and the ability to predict. The learning thrust for this level of research as well as for this level of practice skill would be directed toward measures of relative risk, the development and use of interval and ratio data, the differentiation between dependent and independent variable relationship, the concepts of and criteria for causality, validity, reliability, sensitivity and specificity. The objective is of course to understand and use the design of investigation, to use terms of science, to be able to identify research objectives, to put boundaries on research problems and to generate hypotheses.

Year four focuses upon synthesis not only in the practice realm and in terms of entering the profession, but also in relation to developing an understanding of the ways in which it is possible and relevant to formulate questions which challenge knowledge in the field. Development of a critical, analytical style of thinking in relation to established views of nursing phenomena is fundamental to acquiring such skills. The level is proportionately more complex by year four. Situation prescription is analogous to identifying and operationalising nursing interventions for problem or solution. In research, of course one always has a primary objective the need to control the situation in order to evaluate utility and productivity. It follows that situation prescribing research would include evaluative research, cohort analysis, clinical trials and classic experimental design. The learning thrust here would be directed towards indicators and measures of the efficacy of interventions on critical analysis, on the variety of models of research and on the linkage of nursing care and nursing problems to the quantified indicators of adequacy, appropriateness, effectiveness and efficiency of action. Support courses include study in areas such as nursing theories, epidemiology and theories of evaluation and desired learning outcomes here would include research literacy. Additional objectives may well centre upon writing a comprehensive research proposal or critiquing a research project. These are also entirely appropriate expectations for the baccalaureate graduate. The four classes of objectives identified by year would result in a baccalaureate level graduate demonstrating research literacy and acquiring the ability to make a constructive contribution as an intelligent consumer. I am here suggesting that the objective at the conclusion of the undergraduate process is research literacy. Research literacy constitutes the ability to use research findings, to be able to assess the validity of a research method and to be able to generate researchable objectives or hypotheses. As a research consumer with some understanding of the research process, baccalaureate nursing graduates will hopefully serve as both role models and change agents in relation to positive attitudes and values where research is concerned. I hasten to add that research literacy must not be confused with research mastery. Mastery of the research process requires opportunity to practice in some depth and with some frequency the process of design and implementation of an investigative project. Graduate students normally have an opportunity to participate in research projects being undertaken by faculty members, and in this way gain practical experience with the research process as a part of their programmes of study. The ability to carry out solo investigations, collaborative investigations and to participate in investigations is required for the career investigator.

In this chapter an attempt has been made to demonstrate the similarities (and differences) between the research process and the clinical problem solving process. Nurses, for the most part, have mastered problem solving, but are frequently intimidated by research. To develop a pragmatic perspective for investigation is considered a critical step toward research literacy and subsequent mastery.

REFERENCES

Dickoff, J., & James, P. (1968). Practice Oriented Research: Part II. *Nursing Research, 17,* 545-554.

Diers, D. (1979). *Research in Nursing Practice,* New York: J.B. Lippincott Co.

Haack, D. (1979). *Statistical Literacy: A Guide to Interpretation,* North Scituate, Mass.: Duxbury Press.

Johnson, W. & Hardin, C. (1962). *Content and Dynamics of Home Visits by Public Health Nurses:* Part 1.

Jones, P. (1979). A Terminology for Nursing Diagnosis, *Advances in Nursing Science, 2,* 65-72.

Polit, P. & Hungler, B. (1978). *Nursing Research,* New York: J.B. Lippincott.

Popham, W.J. (1975). *Educational Evaluation,* Englewood Cliffs: Prentice- Hall.

Sackett, D. et al. (1974). The Burlington Randomized Trial of the Nurse Practitioner: Health

Outcomes of Patients, *Annals of Internal Medicine, 80(2)*, 137-142.

Chapter Nine

THE RELATIONSHIP BETWEEN GRADUATE TEACHING AND RESEARCH IN NURSING

Moyra Allen

It is through graduate study in masters' and doctoral programs that students learn to be scholars
and scientists. Here they come to value the content and methods of science in developing their
practice and in pursuing problems which require
investigation. To this end faculty in graduate
programs prepare curricula and select teaching
methods to enable students to augment their clinical expertise, carry out research, evolve theory
and build science. We may surmise that the more
faculty are prepared to involve themselves and
participate in each of these dimensions of the
scientific endeavour, the more their teaching will
reflect the nature of science and the role of the
scientist. The range and scope of graduate teaching and research in a school reflects the preparation and diversity of interests and abilities of
faculty, the development of the associated clinical
nursing and health care services, and the contextu-
al support for research and graduate study. The
interactive nature of the relationship between
graduate teaching and research is crucial to the
development of science. The production of nursing
scientists and the growth of nursing science suf-
fers where graduate teaching and research are
pursued as separate domains and where the pursuit
of science content is other than nursing relevant.
The relationship between graduate teaching and
research in nursing reflects developments in the
nature of health work and the changing function and
expanding role of nursing in the provision of
health care services. There are points in our
short but evolving research history when the changing pattern of this relationship becomes evident.
The first section of this chapter examines the
relationship between graduate teaching and research

in nursing at these critical points. The second part suggests the shape of this relationship for the future if we are to produce scholars and scientists who will build the science which nursing requires to realise its potential in the health care system. Although this chapter is directed to the Canadian scene, it assumes a somewhat similar set of trends in nursing in the U.S., particularly in the beginning stage. The relationship between graduate teaching and research in nursing will be examined in three time periods - pre 1965, between 1965 and 1980, and post 1980.

The following chart portrays the general emphasis in graduate teaching and research in each of these time periods.

Period	Graduate Teaching	Research in Nursing
Pre-1965	Masters' programs for teachers and administrators	Problem solving Descriptive Evaluative
1965-1980	Masters' program with clinical specialisation	Application of knowledge from other disciplines Descriptive Evaluative
Post 1980	Graduate programs oriented to nursing	Seeking knowledge from problems and situations arising in practice Scientific approach

PRE 1965

The scope of nursing has continued to expand throughout this century. In the early years the role of the nurse was reasonably well defined encompassing the traditional function attributed to Florence Nightingale as the founder of modern nursing. With the increasing specificity of medical care, nursing began to incorporate an additional function derivative of the medical plan. The content of this function increased tremendously with the proliferation of medical specialties. With this expansion the work of the nurse became

more prescriptive and aligned with medicine particularly in acute care settings. The ensuing complexity of nursing required nurses to have more
knowledge and be able to master the growing tech-
nologies involved in patient care. Nurse teachers
and administrators with advanced preparation were
required to develop new curricula and to manage
modern nursing services.

As there was no master's program in existence in Canada prior to 1959, nurses sought
further education in the United States undertaking
programs oriented to teaching, administration, and
public health. At that time in Canada the post-RN
baccalaureate program performed a similar function,
preparing teachers, administrators, and public
health nurses. In most cases faculty were themselves prepared in public health, education or
administration. Involvement of faculty in nursing
centered around their leadership roles in professional organisations and in teaching. However,
there was probably a closer relationship between
public health nursing faculty and the practice
field as students were introduced to a new 'clinical discipline'. A few individual faculty members
in other fields (nursing of children, maternity and
psychiatric) were engaged with students in clinical
practice. In general, the emphasis in nursing was
on the application of principles resulting in
procedures, protocols, and programs believed to be
beneficial to the patient, family, or group concerned: such as nursing care related to medical
and surgical treatment plans; prenatal programs and
well-baby clinics delivering the best information
of the day; and nursing care patterned on the
prevailing psychotherapeutic regime of the unit or
institution. Where clinical content was included,
it was derived as a logical deduction from the
medical plan or public health program.

Research was viewed primarily as a method of
problem solving focusing on procedures for the
collection of data to aid in the solution of practical problems in administration and education
(Henderson, 1956). Time and motion studies which
concentrated on the quantity of nursing rather than
the quality, were common (How to Study, 1954; Head
Nurse Study in Canada, 1954). Furthermore, nurses
were relatively certain that their practices were
valuable and that benefits would accrue to patients
and clients who complied with the prescribed protocol and its procedures. From their perspective the
research method was viewed as a way to demonstrate
the value of a program or a procedure, for example

the evaluation of prenatal or other public health programs (American Nurses' Foundation, 1960). Data collection tools - questionnaire and interview, took precedence over the relevance and significance of the problem and issues of design. This approach to research failed to locate the process within the context of science and instead served more to satisfy the biases of faculty and students.

In this era, it was usual for faculty to supervise students' research projects but not to participate in either nursing practice or research themselves. They acted not as models for either nursing or research, but as traditional teachers. In general, research problems for study did not arise from practice nor were they in most instances nursing or health related. Social scientists carried out the large scale research projects of that era, investigating, for the most part, the attributes and characteristics of nurses (Hughes, 1958).

1965 - 1980

With advances in social science and more extensive education for nurses at both the baccalaureate and master's levels, new perspectives emerged as to the nature of nursing and the role of the nurse. One perspective became embodied in the move toward clinical specialisation. The second perspective capitalised on the increasingly popular notion of process in the sciences: growth and development, adaptation, dynamics, systems theory, evolution, etc. To some extent these perspectives were antithetical:

-       specialisation providing a vertical structure; each discrete section with its own unique body of disease-related knowledge from the biological, social and medical sciences; colleagueship with other health care professionals in the specialty services; research questions related to the application of knowledge from other disciplines in nursing (See, 1977).

-       development, process and change notions providing a horizontal structure applicable in all types of situations: individuals, groups, communities, institutions, etc.; knowledge - broad conceptual models; colleagueship with nurses across clinical fields concerned in practice with for example: process ideas as related to the nurse-patient relationship and the implications for nursing of human growth and development; research questions arising out of these new perspectives in practice (Diers & Leonard, 1966).

This general perspective of development failed to compete with the more unique and particular features of clinical specialisation. It was some time before nursing could exchange its vertical paradigm of medical specialties and disease conditions for the more general horizontal model characteristic of all people and all situations. It seemed during this time as though nursing was advancing toward associate specialist status with medicine in the various clinical fields in hospital, in family and group practice, and in public health and primary health care services.

In the United States clinical specialisation reached a peak in which most of the specialties had their counterpart in nursing. This direction to developments in nursing was supported by a similar pattern in the expansion of masters' programs throughout the country. Masters' programs included clinical practice and the incorporation of the body of knowledge relevant to the clinical specialty including social sciences (Gortner & Nahm, 1977). Students learned to master the knowledge and skills of nursing associated with most of the major health and medical problems of the field. Clinical work tended to be hospital-based although efforts were made to extend the nurse's expertise in rehabilitation and prevention. Some faculty practiced nursing in conjunction with their work with students in the clinical field. This approach to nursing provided the scientific knowledge base of the clinical specialty from which to derive a rational set of practices for nursing. The flaw in this method of assessing the requirements for nursing in the disease conditions of a particular specialty is that it results in a set of practices determined *a priori* regardless of the patient or client for whom the nurse is caring. It results in a universal program of nursing generated by the disease condition.

Research investigations revolved around the evaluation of the utility and benefits to be derived from the application of knowledge and theories from other disciplines to the practice of nursing in particular clinical fields. Methodological excellence and technological expertise were of growing concern (See, 1977). A recent analysis of research from 1952 on in *Nursing Research* documents the increasing number of clinical studies headed by the medical-surgical specialties during this period (Brown, Tanner & Padrick, 1984). Research studies in graduate programs and articles in the research journals displayed the profession's growth and sophistication in that most objective of criteria - the manipulation of numbers. The clinical value of significant statistical findings was of less concern than the rigor of the analytical procedures. The contribution to nursing knowledge of such research has been questioned. As late as 1982 the editor of *Nursing Research*, commenting on the supremacy of method over content, wrote:

> I have been astounded by the incredible amount of time and effort that is often spent on mundane work, which is methodologically impeccable while at the same time devoid of substantive content (Downs, 1982).

University schools of nursing in Canada escaped such extensive specialisation in their programs owing to a more broadly based health care system, fewer such highly specialised nurse clinicians, and the time lag in the development of masters' programs.

Post-1980

Over the past few years the right to health has come to be claimed by much of society. The first steps in this direction were taken by the federal government with hospitalisation and, somewhat later, medical care insurance under the philosophy of comprehensiveness, universality, accessibility and availability of health care services. In addition there has been a growing demand by the public for a broad range of services directed toward health and well-being. The strength of the consumer movement has assured greater participation by citizens in these developments. It is believed that with the new Canada Health Act of 1984, there will be opportunity for the provinces to provide insured services for other health care professionals. In the future they too may participate in the expansion of health services. The role of nursing has been changing rapidly to incorporate the goal of health promotion as a central thrust in its practice. With the increase in services directed toward health, the work of the nurse is expanding to include the developmental aspects of healthy living. The opportunity for nursing to play a more comprehensive and responsible role in society's health is now available. Already the increasing number of nurses with graduate degrees and clinical specialisation are making claims for nursing - the value of its service and the expertise it has to offer in the health care field. This movement is accompanied by efforts to identify the components of nursing and to separate the practice of nursing out from other types of professional practice in the health care field. Major attempts are being made to clarify the *persona* of nursing as well as to establish an updated version of nursing in the public mind.

The goal of health promotion with its long-term perspective and family base has given the process and developmental theme, as identified previously, much greater credence in nursing. This emphasis is seen clearly as it is applied to healthful living throughout the lifespan and to the process elements of the nurse-client relationship in health work. This growing acceptance has been supported by the belief in research-based practice, not only as the foundation for the individual nurse's development in the assessment, action, evaluation process, but in the movement of the profession itself to full-fledged legitimacy and autonomy in the health care field. As a result the content of nursing is gaining an identity and is beginning to pervade the study and practice of nursing across all programs and fields.

Evidence is accumulating to show that the nursing component of clinical specialties in graduate programs is becoming increasingly similar. This trend can be seen in the Guidelines for Graduate Education of the Canadian Association of University Schools of Nursing (1980) and earlier in the Characteristics of Graduate Education prepared by the National League for Nursing (1979). A perusal of calendars and bulletins describing masters' programs indicates that specialties are described in more general terms with less well-defined boundaries. In many programs content issues are explored jointly across specialties. The study of nursing itself is becoming the target of our programs as the goals of nursing become more substantial and attain a degree of clarity and as theories of nursing delineate the nature of nursing and its constituent parts and relationships. This trend fosters a search for new approaches to the categorization of clinical specialties. It is as though previously the context for nursing was in relief and became the major focus of a program, for example, children with orthopaedic conditions or patients in a coronary care unit. Now nursing is in relief and we are seeking ways to study it more intensively and in greater depth in the various locales in which nursing goes on.

This concentration on nursing over the past few years has produced a number of theorists, model builders, paradigm makers, and conceptual framers each of whom strives to capture the essence of nursing and to describe its make-up. For the most part their theses have been offered to all clinical fields as frameworks for the practice of nursing. Each perspective may be viewed as an all-purpose version of nursing applicable anywhere nursing is practiced. Thus the basis and rationale for clinical specialisation as previously envisioned no longer holds. With this new prominence of nursing *qua* nursing, we can expect a sharper and more delimited definition of that which is research in nursing.

Research is less concerned now with the application of knowledge from other disciplines in the solution of nursing problems. Rather, the focus is to build knowledge from the investigation of situations within the framework of a particular view or theoretical perspective in nursing. To make progress in this search for knowledge, theorists and researchers are taking the initiative to implement their ideas in the actual practice of nursing. For this reason faculty and their clinical associates are involved with the practice-research continuum as participants. Faculty are no longer able to maintain the armchair stance of their predecessors. Concomitant changes may be noted in the graduate programs across this country with the emphasis on the practice of nursing, whatever the version, and on research. This movement has the potential to change the critical relationships which students develop: from the student as a member of the multidisciplinary clinical team in a specialty to the student as a colleague with faculty in the investigation of particular nursing situations. Not only must faculty practice and investigate nursing but also be knowledgeable of the sciences relevant to the context within which they are working. Graduate teaching cannot be divorced from research; in fact, the content of graduate teaching must now have its own research base.

A recent analysis of nursing literature published in major journals revealed an increasing number of studies in the clinical specialties and some in broader fields such as gerontology and community health. Many more studies were centered around prevention/health promotion and chronic illness/rehabilitation. The authors write:

> With regard to general care orientation of these clinical studies, there has been a shift in emphasis from 1970 to 1980, away from acute illness (from 56% to 20%) toward prevention and health promotion (from 13% to 35%). Such a shift would be in accord with the professed interest of nurses in 'wellness' (Brown, Tanner & Padrick, 1984).

Despite the broader range of studies, a number of inadequacies were cited in the same article: insufficient conceptualisation; scarcity of longitudinal work; primacy of questionnaire and interview techniques, participant observation and unobtrusive measures - a rarity; and measuring tools from other disciplines bearing only loose correspondence to the conceptual meaning of the variables of interest to nursing. It is noteworthy that no study samples families and few events or organisations.

SHAPING THE RELATIONSHIP BETWEEN GRADUATE TEACHING AND RESEARCH

This section addresses some of the critical issues to be considered in shaping the relationship between graduate teaching and research if the potential of nursing is to be realised in society. It is through the complex interplay of practice, research and theory building that faculty and graduate students together are able to add bits of knowledge relevant to nursing in their setting. To the extent that the relationship between graduate teaching and research is exploited, it impacts on the school's own curriculum for the basic preparation of nurses and on the immediate health care delivery system. This relationship will be more generative of faculty and student development and of real knowledge of nursing once its potential is recognised.

Although practice, research and theory enter into each level of university teaching - baccalaureate, master's and doctoral - the emphasis on each differs by program (CAUSN, 1980).

At the baccalaureate level the emphasis is on practice, the student learning to nurse across situations which, in total, encompass the majority of critical variables to which nurses must respond. Research and investigative methods enter largely through the problem posing and problem solving implied in the nursing process and through courses in the other disciplines utilising similar methods such as those in epidemiology, psychology, etc. The theory equivalent may be found in the existing body of knowledge relevant to nursing, but also in the student's own tentative hypothesising of relationships amongst variables across situations.

At the master's level the emphasis is on the method of studying problems in the practice of nursing, that is, the method of research. The practice aspect of nursing is expanded through increased perception and awareness of questions arising in clinical nursing and through the implementation of findings from the student's own investigations and those of others. Students begin to piece together their ideas and to build their own model of nursing. Knowledge from their investigations and those of others contribute to the model. Theoretical positions of other nurses begin to have meaning and relevance for masters' level students.

At the doctoral level the emphasis is on the process of building theory in nursing. The practice and research aspects are furthered through the intensive investigation of one particular clinical nursing problem. The knowledge gained through this process contributes to the student's model of nursing and, with elaboration, to the theory of nursing.

Support for research in nursing has been augmented in university schools by virtue of the increasingly rigorous tenure regulations of universities and by the publish or perish phenomenon. With the economic squeeze of the 80's, resources for research are less available and the resulting competition for funds is generating a new set of influences on the development of nursing research. A school may opt for research at any cost, resulting in a multitude of small unrelated studies. Often the problems for investigation in nursing reflect insufficient exploration characteristic of impoverished practice and methods which fail to meet the requirements of external validity. This approach neither contributes to the discipline of nursing in any significant fashion nor does it support the development of faculty and students. Rather, a concerted effort to mount a program of

research related to the school's goals and directions should be entertained. Guidelines for Graduate Education in Nursing of the Canadian Association of University Schools of Nursing suggest the
following direction:

It is also expected that schools will have
identified a profile of nursing incorporating
the essential ingredients of practice which
faculty believe will convey optimum benefits to
society. This model epitomizes faculty's
philosophy of nursing in its most unique and
elementary form. From this profile faculty
paint a picture of the nurse their educational
programs aim to prepare. Subsumed within the
practice model is the fundamental science or
knowledge base which dictates discipline content (CAUSN, 1980).

The search for discipline content becomes
embodied in the major research program of the
school. The critical questions posed delimit the
sphere of research activity and direct the lines of
inquiry. In this fashion questions requiring
longitudinal investigation and other cross section-
al study provide for continuity and a cumulative
framework. At the moment some faculties follow a
more structured path than others in this pursuit,
but there is no doubt that highly individualised
schools of thought on nursing are developing in
university schools of nursing and their associated
health care agencies across both the United States
and Canada. Such pluralism enriches the field of
inquiry and promotes diversity of direction and
approach in research. This approach to research
reaffirms the importance of the relevance of a
school's programs to its society and of the relat-
edness of its research and investigative efforts in
further expanding the knowledge base for its programs. To the extent that faculty and graduate
students participate together in the research
enterprise will students comprehend the interplay
between practice and research and teaching and
integrate this perspective in their own work.
        In this critical period in the development of
nursing research, the kinds of choices we make are
crucial: the kinds of research we do, the problems
we study and the nature of the theory we build. In
the following section these questions will be
considered more specifically in relation to the
context within which nursing is developing in
Canada.

First, it is important for university schools to identify clearly those factors which should motivate their research and theory building activities. Needless to say, motivation which stems from university tenure policies or from a compulsion to imitate other disciplines will not suffice. Rather, motivation should be generated by the search for knowledge upon which to predict and control the outcomes of practice so as to influence the health of people in predictable ways. To the extent that the practice of nursing is based on real knowledge, nursing is able to be accountable and to accept responsibility for its practice. It is only through this pursuit that an enlarged role for nursing can be legitimised within the health care system.

The type of knowledge we seek through research is dictated by our conception of nursing and its goals within the health care system. The overall goal of health promotion for nursing has been proclaimed by the Canadian Nurses Association most recently in its presentations to the Minister in view of the proposed amendments to the Canada Health Act during 1983-84 (Canadian Nurses Association, 1984). This position was earlier affirmed by Verna Splane in her address to the Canadian Association of University Schools of Nursing when she said that nursing is the profession best fitted at this time to deal with the primary health care of people (Splane, 1982). This means the everyday business of health and well-being of people whether sick and in hospital or sick or well in the home or other location in the community. It is important to recall that Florence Nightingale in her *Notes on Nursing* described the function of nursing in health oriented terms in 1859:

> The very elements of what constitutes good nursing are as little understood for the well as for the sick. The same laws of health or of nursing, for they are in reality the same, obtain among the well as among the sick (p. 6).

> And nothing but observation and experience will teach us the ways to maintain or to bring back the state of health (p. 74).

> And what nursing has to do in either case (medicine & nature), is to put the patient in the best condition for nature to act upon him (p. 75).

Later, Isabel M. Stewart also described Florence Nightingale's notion of nursing in terms of health promotion:

Miss Nightingale was not interested in simply keeping people alive. She insisted that one must live in order to be well. Well-being is impossible unless one has the means for living -- the proper environment, freedom to grow and enjoy life. Nursing is helping people to live (1943, p. 48).

If nurses in general and our university schools of nursing in particular concur with this view of nursing as the practice of health promotion, then the knowledge base we are seeking is the science of health promoting interactions (Pugnaire, 1981), or more broadly the science of health promoting situations (Warner, 1980). With this research direction for nursing clearly formulated, some specific questions about basic research and applied research follow. Basic research revolves around the question of health (Allen, 1982).

What are the attributes of healthy families?

What are the attributes of successful coping and healthy development in varying sorts of life situations and states - interpersonal dynamics, coping styles, resources, goals, outcomes, etc.?

What is the picture of development in healthy families?

How do children, adults, and aged persons, and persons in various stages of acute and chronic illness, learn and acquire healthful behaviors?

What are some of the early signs of healthy behavior in a new family? Of less healthy behavior?

What is the context within which healthy families arise? Less healthy families?

Applied research focuses on the ways and means of health promotion:

How can nursing foster the development of healthy families in varying sorts of life situations and states?

Other disciplines in addition to nursing are now engaged in studying the attributes of healthy people and, at the same time, building a concept of health. At this point in the development of nursing knowledge and nursing research considerable exploratory and descriptive research of a qualitative nature is required. Nursing is and can be engaged in this work at many levels - individual, family/group and community - and in a wide variety of situations - new families, aging people, chronic illness, and so on. It is prudent that nursing concentrates on situations of which it has particular knowledge and skills as well as easy access to study populations. Furthermore, it would seem that the selection of situations critical to society in view of their need for health would generate more visible and immediate benefits.

A crucial first step in research in a professional discipline is to describe in detail the situations professionals deal with - in the case of nursing, varying states of being healthy and the process that leads thereto. To date we describe these situations through the diagnostic labels we apply, but they tend to be at a gross and general level and are often disease-related. Once we evolve theory which accounts for the process of people being and becoming healthy we shall be in a position to label and classify the sorts of situations which confront nurses in their practice. In the meantime each school should identify the descriptive diagnostic or assessment labels they are now using to ensure that they are congruent with the theory or framework faculty espouse in the teaching of nursing.

Situations must be created for faculty and students in graduate programs to work with patients/clients/families in seeking those which are health producing. Owing to the dearth of information on the health promoting process, it is important that students as well as clients view their activities within a discovery framework. Here faculty member, student and client are engaged overtime in an exploratory endeavor - seeking information, gathering evidence, trying out, validating, modifying, experimenting, etc. Nurse and client are engaged in a joint inquiry and scientific venture. The price is high and the requirements demanding for faculty: practice, teaching, scholarship, research, university and community affairs, and leadership in the profession. The traditional view of the researcher as an individual generating research questions based on self interest and working independently is no longer valid. The practice-research continuum is a necessity if research work is to be reality-based in the practice of health promotion.

Students must be socialised in their graduate programs into the practice of nursing and the study and investigation of nursing as inseparable components in their career development (Allen, Cox & Parker, 1979). This socialisation process could be accomplished most effectively through the development of *centres of nursing* both in the hospital and in the larger community, settings which provide for both academic and clinical faculty to engage in practice, education and research directed toward a particular set of health care needs with which nursing is concerned. It is through such an endeavor that the achievement of a unique and valued service would eventually augment the visibility of nursing in the setting and in the nursing community. The knowledge nursing seeks through research is a joint venture of nurse and client, teacher and student.

NOTES

1. Masters' programs in Nursing were started at the University of Western Ontario in 1959 and McGill University in 1961.

REFERENCES

Allen, M. (1982). A model of nursing: A plan for research and development. In *International Conference Proceedings: Research - A Base for the Future?* (pp. 315-330). Edinburgh: Nursing Studies Research Unit, University of Edinburgh.

Allen, M., Cox, B. & Parker, N. (1979). *Doctoral education in nursing. In The Proceedings on Doctoral Preparation for Canadian Nurses: Ph.D. Nursing.* Ottawa: Canadian Nurses Association.

American Nurses Foundation (1960). Pathway to future progress in nursing care. *Nursing Research, 9*, 4-7.

Brown, J., Tanner, C., & Padrick, K. (1984). Nursing's search for scientific knowledge. *Nursing Research, 33*, 26-32.

Canadian Association of University Schools of Nursing (1980). *Guidelines for graduate education in nursing leading to a master's degree*. Ottawa: Author.

Canadian Nurses Association (1984). CNA connection. *The Canadian Nurse, 80*, 6.

Diers, D.T., & Leonard, R.C. (1966). Interaction analysis in nursing research. *Nursing Research, 15*, 225-228.

Downs, F. (1982). Editorial. *Nursing Research, 31*, 4.

Gortner, S., & Nahm, H. (1977). An overview of nursing research in the United States. *Nursing Research, 26*, 10-33.

Henderson, V. (1956). Research in nursing practice: When? (Editorial). *Nursing Research, 4*, 99.

How to Study the Nursing Activities in a Patient Unit (1954). Washington, D.C.: United States Public Health Service.

Hughes, E. (1958). *20,000 nurses tell their story*. Philadelphia: J.B. Lippincott.

National League for Nursing (1979). Characteristics of graduate education in nursing leading to the master's degree. *Nursing Outlook, 27(3)*, 206.

Nightingale, F. (1859). *Notes on nursing: What it is and what it is not*. London: Harrison & Sons. (facsimile reproduced by J.B. Lippincott)

Pugnaire, C. (1981). *The science of health - promoting interactions - A theoretical perspective*. Montreal: McGill University School of Nursing.

See, E. (1977). The ANA and research in nursing. *Nursing Research, 26*, 165.

Splane, V. (1982). Fashioning the future. *Nursing Papers, 16(3),* 12-24.

Stewart, I. (1943). *The education of nurses: Historical foundations and modern trends.* New York: MacMillan.

Warner, M. (1980). *Notes on health - Promoting situations.* Montreal: School of Nursing, McGill University.

Chapter Ten

RESEARCH TRAINING AND FUNDING FOR NURSES IN THE UNITED KINGDOM

Jack C. Hayward
Sylvia R. Lelean

INTRODUCTION

Many of the reforms of nursing instigated by Florence Nightingale were based upon data which were carefully collected and skillfully analysed. Nevertheless, the new system of nurse training did not include any element of research training to develop such a capacity within the profession. Undoubtedly, Florence Nightingale possessed flair and initiative, qualities which appear to have been notably lacking in the nursing leadership at the end of the nineteenth century; so much so that Simpson (1971) commented that 'the spirit of enquiry had been effectively checked.'

It is unwise, however, to single out nursing as a special case for criticism, because, during the latter half of the last century, few professions had established either the acceptability or relevance of research to the practitioner. Perhaps surprisingly, this was true also of many universities, for, in 1852, the long-established and much-respected universities of Oxford and Cambridge fiercely resisted the idea of research being part of the educational process and told a Royal Commission that 'research would promulgate infidelity and scepticism' (Ashby, 1974). By 1900, however, the established professions such as medicine and veterinary science were creating a recognised research base, a development which often ran parallel to the establishment of university degrees in those subjects. Whilst these universities had a tradition of awarding the 'higher' research degrees of Doctor of Science (D.Sc.) and Doctor of Literature (D. Litt.), pressure was being put upon them during the early part of the century to award also the 'lower' research degree of Doctor of Philosophy (Ph.D.) in order to attract more students, especially from the United States of America. Oxford awarded its first Ph.D. degree in 1917 while London held out until 1920 when, finally, as Simpson (1983) remarked:

> The Ph.D. arrived in all British universities: symbol of the modern era of organised training in research -- conceived and nurtured in Germany, imported and commercialised by America and finally introduced into Britain in order to wean the latter's students away from the former's universities (p. 159).

Research thereby became an accepted post-graduate activity in many disciplines, but not in nursing. As well as resisting the Ph.D. degree, London University also resisted the establishment of a Chair in Nursing. This was something for which Mrs. Ethel Bedford Fenwick (1857-1947) fought long and hard, in addition to founding the International Council of Nurses in 1903 and working for the enactment of State Registration of Nurses in 1919 (Hector, 1973). In fact it took until 1977 before London University established its first Chair in Nursing Studies, something which Oxford, Cambridge, and many other Universities have not yet seen fit to do.

There seems little doubt that the strong links developed during the early 1900's between the established professions and British Universities set a pattern for education and research to develop side by side and that this pattern influenced research opportunities and funding. Hence, nursing, being outside of these seminal developments, made little progress in research for the first half of the century, nor did it establish a meaningful presence in the universities until the 1960's (Hayward, 1982). The founding of nursing departments in institutions of higher education may therefore be seen as a 'key to the research door'.

It may thus be useful to examine briefly the main sources of funds available for research in the United Kingdom (U.K.) and the kinds of access nurses have to such monies before turning to the training of nurses as researchers. Research into nursing can be viewed as part of the broader spectrum of health services research which has three main sources of funds. First, the 'dual-support' system administered through the University Grants Committee (UGC) and Research Councils; second, through direct support from Government Departments; and third, from private funding sources including charities.

RESEARCH FUNDING

The Dual Support System

The University Grants Committee, which is comprised of academics, has the responsibility of distributing money provided by government to the universities. It contributes to essential academic services such as university libraries and accommodation and facilities such as laboratories. Salaries for tenured academic teaching posts are funded by the UGC; hence, the decision to fund teaching posts in university departments of nursing was of critical importance to the development of nursing research, because a university teacher is expected to devote a substantial amount of time to research to advance his/her subject and to benefit the university and himself/herself. To achieve academic respectability in the eyes of established disciplines, nursing academics must fulfil such expectations, which, to a certain degree, has been the case in the United Kingdom. For the first time, therefore, in nursing education, research was seen not merely as desirable but essential. Of course, for the UGC to fund such posts presupposes that there are universities willing and able to house such initiatives and a steady supply of students of sufficient academic calibre to benefit from undergraduate and post-graduate work. Happily, in the U.K. both the former (albeit initially with a certain reluctance) and the latter (most university degree courses in nursing are over-subscribed by applicants of high academic quality) requirements have been fulfilled. In contrast to the situation in North America, though, the proportion of student nurses undertaking baccalaureate level preparation comprises less than five percent of the total (Hayward, 1982). Because of the complexities inherent in the system, calculating the precise research resource represented by approximately fifty teaching posts (estimate for 1983) in university nursing departments funded by the UGC is problematic, but it nevertheless represents a definite and long-term facility.

The Research Councils collectively administer the largest source of non-industrial research monies in the U.K. These are for the well-established areas of Agriculture and Food (AFRC),

Medicine (MRC), Natural Environment (NERC), Science and Engineering (SERC) and the Social Sciences (SSRC) recently renamed the Economic and Social Research Council (ESRC). Research Councils are funded by the Department of Education and Science, the allocation of funds being decided with advice from the Advisory Board for the Research Councils.

The MRC and ESRC both fund research of direct or indirect relevance to nursing. The MRC's major focus, though, is on bio-medical research with only a small proportion of its budget allocated to health services research. Both Councils support the training of researchers in their relevant disciplines and offer a range of post graduate awards mainly through appropriate university departments or in designated research units. To date, very little research into nursing has been funded by the MRC or ESRC, nor have many nurses applied for such funding. One reason may be that, as yet, few nurses have sufficient research experience to compete successfully for an award from these bodies.

Government Departments
Since 1972, research commissioned by Government Departments has conformed to the 'customer-contractor' principle (i.e., 'the customer says what he wants; the contractor does it (if he can); and the customer pays') as recommended in the Rothschild report on government-funded research (1972). Because of the urgent need to understand more about nursing, essentially for practical and policy reasons rather than theoretical analysis, the majority of nursing research in the U.K. has been funded by Government Health Departments.[1]

The DHSS administers in the region of 11 million pounds per annum on health services research of which nursing has about a six percent share. Most of this research is commissioned through Research Liaison Groups (RLG) which provide an opportunity for policy makers, research managers, external scientific advisers and service advisers to work together on identifying priorities and commissioning research (Kogan & Henkel, 1983). Research Liaison Groups exist for most client groups, e.g. the elderly, mentally handicapped. The Nursing RLG was set up in 1973 under the Chairmanship of the Chief Nursing Officer. Its brief includes the development of research in nursing which incorporates research training, the dissemination of information about research, the

development of research centres as well as commissioning research in nursing education, service and
practice (Lelean, 1980).

The National Health Service itself funds a
relatively small amount of research. In an attempt
to decentralise a proportion of research funding
from central government to Regional Health Authorities, the Locally Organised Research (LOR) scheme
was introduced in 1975. Through this scheme, the
fourteen Regions in England support local research
initiatives, which are open to applications from
any health service discipline. The LOR scheme thus
represents an advance on the previous decentralised
clinical research provision which was solely for
medical research. The LOR scheme enables nurses
working in the NHS to obtain grants for research
expenses. Applications are considered by grant
awarding committees and some degree of research
expertise is expected. Applications which incorporate training in research methods for a nurse would
need, therefore, to be made in the name of an
experienced researcher. In spite of early teething
troubles, a few nursing projects have now been
funded in this way, most being concerned with
issues arising from service responsibilities.

Private Funding Sources

Charitable organisations have a well-established
tradition of contributing to medical research in
the United Kingdom. Most, however, have confined
their interests to areas such as cancer, heart
disease or, in more recent times, long-term inca-
pacitating illnesses such as multiple sclerosis.
In recent years, certain charities have come to
realise that nursing is equally worth supporting
and a start has been made by the funding of a few
fellowships and studentships for nurses. It is
often the case that, once a precedent has been
established, others follow, so that, in future
years, charitable support may constitute an important resource for nursing research.

RESEARCH TRAINING

Overview

As with any skilled activity, research methods and
techniques are initially best learned and applied
in a suitable environment and with adequate

supervision. In the universities, this is achieved by post-graduate study at various levels, such students often being supported financially by grants from research councils, especially in science and medicine. Taught courses to Masters level and research degrees of Master of Philosophy (M Phil), Doctor of Philosophy (Ph.D.), together with post-doctoral research funded by Research Councils or charities comprise the mainstream of scientific research training in the U.K. It has become clear, however, that wide variations exist between institutions in the way in which, for example, a Ph.D. course is followed; some departments focus entirely on the production of an original piece of work leading to a thesis with almost no requirement that taught courses be attended; others have a sizable, though rarely examined, taught component. For the majority, therefore, knowledge of research methods is restricted to those applicable to the thesis topic though this knowledge may be at a very advanced level. It is likely that most students working within a discipline will tend to focus on one main method, such as survey techniques, action research or experimental design to the virtual exclusion of other approaches. In no way can this be seen as a comprehensive training in research methods and may not serve the best interests of either the student or the discipline.

This, and similar questions were considered by the Working Party on Post-Graduate Education (1982) set up by the Advisory Board for the Research Councils. Although its terms of reference were restricted to science and social science students, many of the issues were relevant to post-graduate education in nursing. The Working Party highlighted problem areas such as research topic selection, the nature and frequency of supervision, individual versus group projects as a form of training, the place of taught courses and whether or not these should be a compulsory and examined part of every Ph.D. programme. Academic institutions were advised that all research students should be given a thorough grounding in research methods, that all research topics should be heavily influenced by staff interests, that wherever possible work should be carried out in groups rather than by isolated individuals, and that there should be frequent contact between supervisors and students. The Research Councils, for their part, were advised that they should take into account the benefits of placing students in large departments and that when deciding upon awards, they should discriminate in favor of those departments which effect the above policies.

For nursing research, the implications of the report are twofold. First, that students should, whenever possible, be encouraged by means of the funding policy to enrol in large departments having established research interests and programmes and where supervision is taken seriously; second, that there are distinct advantages in working with a group of people with common research interests, where the resultant Ph.D. makes a contribution to an overall programme. The Working Party states that 70 per cent of scientific research is now carried out in this way (para. 250).

Research Training for Nurses

Two main points emerge from an overview of research in nursing in the United Kingdom. First, with little more than 20 years of development behind it, such research is still in its infancy with regard to its base, personnel and track record. Second, the range of activities encompassed by the term nursing is so broad that, as with medicine, no single method or theoretical framework is likely to be universally applicable to the potentially wide range of research questions which may arise. Central premises exist, of course, and there may well be broad agreement as to what nurses are attempting to do for patients or society in general. Without loss of perspective, therefore, examination of other emergent disciplines may provide nursing with useful pointers. For example 'a' theory human behavior, or 'a' theory of learning are rarely spoken of these days. Rather, the trend has been to look at human responses and activities in discrete and circumscribed areas and to study them using a variety of methods.

Once the need for research as a contribution to nursing knowledge is accepted, the immediate problem becomes one of preparing a cadre of researchers with skills to examine the tremendous breadth of activities which constitute nursing. These range from acute surgery and intensive therapy on the one hand, to the care of the mentally handicapped on the other, and the almost infinite variety of roles and responsibilities lying between. In the U.K. with less than five percent of all registered nurses holding a first (baccalaureate) degree and even fewer with a post-graduate qualification in research, the task of preparing such a pool of expertise is, indeed, daunting.

The first known funding of research training for nurses dates back to 1953 when Boots Pharmaceuticals awarded research fellowships to nurses to study at the University of Edinburgh and who, subsequently, acquired Ph.D. degrees. However, it was not until the late 1960's that there was any attempt to prepare systematically nurses in this way. In 1967, two initiatives were spearheaded from DHSS in London which had important and far-reaching consequences for nurses in the U.K. These were the setting up of the Study of Nursing Care research project and the establishment of the Nursing Research Fellowship scheme.

The Study of Nursing Care project was based at the Royal College of Nursing (RCN) in London and was set up in response to a perceived need to develop measures of the quality of nursing care to be used in the determination of nurse manpower requirements. Because nurses trained and experienced in research were not available to undertake the work, the project provided instruction and supervision for nurse research assistants. These nurses worked under the guidance of a steering group comprising experienced researcher workers from the medical and social sciences and under the direction of a nurse project leader (McFarlane, 1970). During the course of the project (1967-1973) twelve nurses received formal training in research methods and carried out a piece of original research. Six obtained either an M. Phil. or Ph.D. degree. This project constituted the first U.K. attempt at an organised approach to research training in nursing and had both an immediate and long term impact. The initial gain was to bring research to the attention of nurses - often for the first time - highlighting that nursing care could and should be critically put under the microscope and that this should be done by nurses themselves. The long term impact resulted from two sources: first, the project conceived 14 publications; the first set the scene, the next twelve examined discrete aspects of nursing care and the last one tried to pull the threads together. These publications were, and are still, used in teaching and practice and other researchers have used the findings in developing further nursing's knowledge. Additionally, many of the research assistants have subsequently taken up posts in higher education, official organisations and the NHS where they may perhaps further influence the training of nurse researchers and the utilisation of research findings.

Research Fellowships
The first Nursing Research Fellowship was awarded
by DHSS in 1967. Since then the scheme has been
modified over time to meet changing needs and
circumstances. The objectives of a fellowship are
to provide suitably qualified and experienced
nurses with the opportunity to acquire a thorough
grounding in the methods of research and to carry
out a systematic study of an aspect of nursing care
of their choosing for a research degree. Through
this scheme, it is hoped to establish a cadre of
nurses who can research nursing practices and help
to spread an appreciation of research throughout
the profession. The scheme has considerable flexibility and nurses can be accepted for full- or
part-time research training in a university or
polytechnic department of their choice - not necessarily a nursing department. When the scheme first
started, two universities agreed to take the research fellows. Gradually, as nurses demonstrated
that they could hold their own alongside other
scholars, this facility was widened to remove
geographical constraints. At present, non-graduate
(diploma) nurses with considerable professional
experience may apply for an award alongside graduate nurses so long as they fulfil the criteria for
acceptance by their chosen university or polytechnic; however, with the increasing number of
graduate nurses now applying, their chance of
getting an award in open competition is becoming
more difficult and the time is fast coming when
this facility will need to be reassessed.
Over the years, the number of applications for
fellowships has increased considerably. In 1967,
one fellowship was awarded. By 1974, sufficient
interest was generated to warrant convening a
selection panel. Every year since, the number of
applications has been rising steadily, until in
1983, fifty nurses applied for awards, of whom nine
were successful. Notwithstanding its success, the
scheme has created certain organisational difficulties. For instance, in 1980 support through the
scheme was available to any nurse of any grade
currently working in higher education, the NHS or
any other organisation. Because of the increasing
demand, not to mention increasing salary awards, it
was recognised that certain restrictions needed to
be introduced to make the best use of the money
available. It was decided therefore to:

1. convert the scheme into one offering research studentships, which title reflects more accurately the true nature of the training awards;

2. restrict awards to nurses working in the NHS or currently undertaking undergraduate degree courses where their employment immediately before degree studies was in the NHS; and

3. restrict the awards to nurses working up to and including senior tutor (education) and senior nurse 6 (clinical) grades (i.e., middle management).

For full-time awards full salary is paid (including increments, superannuation and national insurance contributions) plus university fees and a specified amount for research expenses. Part-time awards are for university fees and research expenses only. To date, one hundred nurses have held, or are holding, these fellowships or studentships. Inevitably, not all have been successful, but the overall success rate of the scheme compares favorably with other groups.

Like those who took part in the Study of Nursing Care project, these nurses are having a long term influence upon the development of research in nursing through their publications and the posts they hold. Approximately one-third hold research posts in university departments, research units, or the NHS; another third hold teaching posts in the NHS or higher education, whilst the remaining third hold clinically oriented posts. Although the foregoing has described developments in England and Wales, both Scotland and Northern Ireland have their own nursing research training schemes funded by the Government Health Departments. Whilst each country is administered at Government level separately, nursing education in the four countries comprising the U.K. is controlled now by one Council[2] with each country having its own National Board to put into effect the education policy. However, the recent introduction, for the first time, of one U.K. register for all nurses facilitates movement between the four countries. Thus each country benefits from each other's scheme.

Research Assistantships
Research training for nurses has been facilitated by
the establishment of an increasing number of departments of nursing in universities and polytechnics.
The first university Department of Nursing was
established in 1957 in the University of Edinburgh
although its Chair in Nursing -- the first in the
U.K. and, indeed, Europe - was not established until
1972. Since then, Chairs in Nursing have been
established in the Universities of Manchester,
London, Surrey and, most recently, Ulster and Wales.
At present there are about twenty-five university or
polytechnic departments of nursing in the U.K.; many
of these are active in research and regularly submit
proposals to grant awarding bodies. If successful,
they will often subsequently employ nurse research
assistants. This is another method by which nurses
can obtain research training and is becoming increasingly important for those not aspiring to a
research degree.

A handful of nursing research units now exist
in the U.K., situated in universities, often as an
integral part of the departments of nursing studies,
professional organisations and the NHS. Once again,
the University of Edinburgh led the way, in 1971.
These units, under the direction of experienced
nurse researchers, are now starting to play their
part in training nurses in research methods, either
through specific fellowships attached to the units
or by employing nurses as research assistants under
the guidance of a project leader. This method of
research training will become increasingly important
as more such units are set up.

Nurses can also get a good grounding in research methods in the multidisciplinary health
service research units funded by the DHSS and SHHD.
At present, these facilities are not exploited
sufficiently, but, often, a research assistant with
nursing expertise has added an essential dimension
to the work of the unit. In addition, the nurse
gains experience in research methods.

Increasingly over the last 10 years, nurses
have taken up appointments as research assistants
(sometimes called research sisters or clinical
research nurses) to medical research workers. There
may still be an element of exploitation in this
arrangement if the nurse is used just as a data
collector who also has some 'medical' knowledge.
Increasingly, though, the nurse becomes an integral
part of the research team, not only making a valuable contribution to the conduct of the research
but, at the same time, learning about clinical

research methods. It is not unknown for these
research nurses to register for a higher degree on
the basis of their own research which is complementary to the main clinical investigation.

In summary, although much as been achieved in
setting up systems whereby nurses can be trained in
research methods, much still needs to be done. The
completion of one research project does not make a
researcher - the newly acquired expertise must be
developed and nurtured as it grows in order that the
profession can eventually benefit from high calibre
research. In addition to examining their own
profession and its work, nurse researchers should
become part of multidisciplinary groups of health
care scientists working on related projects connect-
ed by a common theme and, to this end, they need to
hone their new-found expertise in the usual cut and
thrust of academic peer review and debate. The main
initiatives in enabling British nurses to obtain
research training have been taken by Government
Health Departments. However, the major responsibility for scientific research training normally falls
to the Research Councils. Both the ESRC and MRC
award research studentships and maybe the younger
graduate nurse interested in research training
should now be seeking support through these funding
bodies.

The only rationale for research activity in
nursing is the improvement of practice, education or
management and, through it, to improve the care
delivered to the patient or client. Thus, another
area which needs continuing attention is the utilisation of research findings, for it is pointless
training nurses to undertake research if the findings are then to lie fallow and not be used.
Professional practice of any kind does not, and
cannot, exist and develop on the basis of research
findings alone. Professions occupy a very privileged position in society by virtue of the public
trust placed in them and it is easy for such groups
to become inward looking and complacent. The
numerous consumer groups and patients' associations
soon remind those in health care when the needs of
the public are not being met. It is incumbent on
the profession itself, however, to monitor and
develop its practice in keeping with changes in the
values and attitudes of any particular society and
to keep pace with scientific and technical progress.

To date, the volume of nursing activities which
has actually been examined or modified by *nursing*
research remains woefully small. Nursing will not
thrive and change to meet new challenges on the

findings of research alone. But, given appropriate
questions and suitable methods and skills on the
part of the nurse researcher, a unique and valuable
contribution can be made to the ever changing art
and science of professional nursing.

NOTES

1. Those concerned are the Department of Health
    and Social Security (DHSS) for England and
    Wales and, to a lesser extent, for Northern
    Ireland, and the Scottish Home and Health
    Department.

2. The United Kingdom Central Council for Nursing,
    Midwifery and Health Visiting.

REFERENCES

Ashby, E. (1974). *Adapting universities to a techno-
    logical society.* London: Jossey-Bass Series in
    Higher Education.

Framework for Government Research and Development
    (1972). (Rothschild Report). Command 5046.
    London: Her Majesty's Stationery Office.

Hayward, J. (1982). Universities and nursing educa-
    tion. *Journal of Advanced Nursing, 7,* 371-377.

Hector, W. (1973). *The work of Mrs. Bedford-Fenwick
    and the rise of professional nursing.* London:
    Royal College of Nursing.

Kogan, M., & Henkel, M. (1983). *Government and
    research - The Rothschild experiment in a
    government department.* London: Heinemann
    Educational Books.

Lelean, S. (1980). Research in nursing: An overview
    of DHSS initiatives in developing research in
    nursing. *Nursing Times, 76*(2), 5-8.

McFarlane, J. (1970). *The proper study of the nurse:
    An account of the first two years of a research
    project "The Study of Nursing Care".* London:
    Royal College of Nursing.

*Report of the Working Party on Postgraduate Educa-
    tion* (1982). (Chairman: Sir P. Swinnerton-

Dyer). London: The Advisory Board for the Research Councils.

Simpson, H.M. (1971). Research in nursing - The first steps. *Nursing Mirror, 132*(11), 22-27.

Simpson, R. (1983). *How the PhD came to Britain - A century of struggle for post graduate education.* Surrey: Society for Research into Higher Education.

PART IV: SELECTED PERSPECTIVES

Chapter Eleven

RESEARCH   DEVELOPMENTS   IN   CLINICAL   SETTINGS: A
CANADIAN PERSPECTIVE

Margaret C. Cahoon

The origins of nursing research are in research in
clinical settings, in the studies of Florence
Nightingale of practice and environmental conditions
(Woodham-Smith, 1950). Nightingale made accurate
clinical observations, recorded them in meticulous
detail, analysed them with statistical sophistication, and reported the results to convince some of
the most influential leaders of the time that
nursing makes an indisputable difference in health
care.
     Without accurate observations and their docu-
mentation, she said, 'we will be useless with all
our devotion' (Nightingale, 1859). The lack of
documentation led her to become a 'passionate
statistician' (Kopf, 1961, p. 388), who had a
'positive genius for marshalling definite knowledge'
(Kopf, 1961, p. 404). She persuaded Sir Francis
Galton to establish the first chair of statistics in
Oxford for she believed that the use of statistics
could influence the health of mankind.
     Nightingale was one of the most intellectually
able, sensitive, courageous and productive scholars
the world has ever known (Schlotfeldt, 1975, p.
180). She left a heritage to nursing, to statistics
and to medicine in drawing attention to the need for
measuring the outcomes of both nursing and medical
care (Nightingale, 1863). She identified the
quintessential focus for nursing research, its
practice, more than a century ago.
     In this chapter the author presents a brief
overview of the revival of nursing research in
clinical settings during the past quarter-century,
identifies the rationale for it, describes strategies that have emerged, specifies some of the major
resources, and indicates some of the supportive and
restraining forces that may influence the

introduction of nursing research into 'natural' field settings. No argument is made in this chapter for the development of a nursing research unit in all clinical settings but inherent is the theme that nurses in all settings must take steps to reduce the present gap between practice and research. This chapter is not in any sense a manual for nursing research development.

The content in this chapter is derived from the author's synthesis of what others have reported in writing and in interviews; her visits to various types of nursing research units in the past decade and participation in the Nursing Research Unit of the Department of Nursing, University of Edinburgh in 1975-76, as the first post-doctoral fellow; and her experiences in the development of the Sunny-brook-University of Toronto Nursing Project as a Bertha Rosenstadt Professor of Research from 1980 to 1982. Less has been written about nursing research development than about any other major change in clinical nursing.

This chapter does not include reference to the research assistant roles undertaken by some nurses assigned to medical research teams to assist in identifying subjects, or to collect and/or process data for medical and psychosocial studies. Nor does it include the roles of nurses in hospital systems analysis/work study groups. Although such experiences were helpful to some in the first generation of nurse researchers in terms of learning how research is done in other practical sciences, because they do not entail responsibility for substantive decisions about research questions and designs involving nursing judgment (Stinson, 1986) they are not central to the development of nursing research in clinical settings.

An Overview of the Revival of Nursing Research in Clinical Settings
Nightingale's exemplary nursing research behaviour did not substantially penetrate either the nursing practice or nursing education systems that were to develop over the next several decades. However, a few studies were done by nurses in the early 1900's, in collaboration with physicians, and in school settings prior to and about the time of the movement of nursing education into the universities in Canada. Also, pressures from nursing educators for improvements in nursing education led to a virtual chain of major educational studies which began in the late 1920's and continued to be a primary focus

of attention for almost half a century in Canada. In these early educational studies nurses collaborated with educators in planning and conducting the investigations, a way of gaining experiential learning that supplemented the kinds of research preparation which some of them were getting in graduate programs in faculties of education.

In 1928 Bertha Harmer, then Director of the School for Graduate Nurses, McGill University and Director of Nursing of the Royal Victoria Hospital, Montreal, began to plan for the development of nursing research in the Royal Victoria Hospital. In 1929 a fellowship was given to a nurse by Dr. C.F. Merton, then Dean of the Faculty of Medicine, McGill University, that enabled her to develop research in one ward over the period of a year's time (Harmer, 1932). Very little about that research has been documented. The early development of nursing research in Notre-Dame Hospital, Montreal, may have been an indirect outcome of Harmer's project (Decary, 1956).

There was a resurgence of interest in clinical nursing studies about 1950 but clinical studies were relatively infrequent in Canada until the late 1960's. A few were done by nurses employed in clinical settings, many of which were done by nurses as part of their degree requirements in graduate programs. The majority of studies were conducted by university nursing faculty members and/or, as of the late 1960's, their graduate students. With few exceptions only a very few nurses continued to do a chain or cluster of related clinical studies. In these studies the researcher entered a clinical setting to collect the data, then returned to academia to analyse the data and prepare the report, a pattern of research activity not conducive to continuity in the study of a major problem area and characteristic of research in the other health sciences.

The development of clinical nursing research in Canada is to some extent directly and indirectly linked with related developments in the United States and in Britain. In the United States the first centre for nursing research was developed at Teachers College, Columbia University, New York, in 1953, with a five-year grant from the Rockefeller Foundation. Its focus was to strengthen and improve education for nursing by conducting research on problems in nursing and nursing education, to disseminate the results of research, and to prepare nurses to conduct research in nursing (Bunge, 1958, p. 113). Although it had been anticipated that problems in nursing practice would be studied, almost all of the research that ensued was in nursing education.

Very shortly afterwards, Harriet Werley developed a nursing research department in the Walter Reed Army Institute of Research (Werley, 1962). This WRAIR research program was established to parallel the units already in existence in medicine, dentistry and veterinary medicine, as well as that of the Army Medical Service Research and Development Command, with its research units in various parts of the world. A decade later Werley reported that, 'Despite [these] unique opportunities ... nursing research did not grow and flourish to the point where nurse researchers generally took their places beside the clinical or field investigators of the other professional disciplines in the Army units' (Werley, 1972, p. 718).

Nevertheless, by 1963 the Veterans Administration developed a policy statement emphasising the responsibility of nurses in leadership positions for creating a climate that would foster a spirit of inquiry and provide a means for nurses to apply the scientific process in the solution of problems, and a position paper which emphasised responsibility for the continued improvement of professional nursing practice through the accumulation of new nursing knowledge (Abrahams, 1968). An organised program of research resulted which included opportunities for formal and experiential learning opportunities in nursing research and for the provision of consultation for nurses involved in research projects.

From the late 1960's a number of major U.S. teaching hospitals established nursing research centres within the nursing departments to provide nurses with the opportunity to conduct scientific investigations to improve the quality of patient care. Several descriptions appear in the literature. For example, Hanson described his experiences in the development of research in nursing service in the Virginia Mason Hospital in Seattle (Hanson, 1971); and Padilla described her approach to the introduction of research in The City of Hope Medical Center (Padilla, 1978). The development of a model for nursing research in the Memorial Sloan-Kettering Cancer Center in New York (Scott, Oberst & Dropkin, 1978) indicates the sophistication of some of these units.

A centre for nursing research was developed at Wayne State University College of Nursing in 1969 by Harriet Werley to plan and develop nursing research projects and to provide an organisational structure

for incorporating the services from other disciplines into nursing research. This development was
followed by the establishment of many similar
nursing research centres or units within faculties
of nursing in the United States (Carnegie, 1978, p.
218), and this movement has continued. These
specialised structures are seen to have had a major
impact upon the development of faculty and upon
student research. However, their effect upon
clinical nursing settings appears to have been quite
variable.

In the sixties, several American* university
nursing faculty members began to have joint appointments in health care agencies, a factor which tended
to result in their research and that of their
graduate students being carried out in a particular
clinical setting. Undoubtedly this movement influenced the further development of nursing research
units in major teaching hospitals and brought
practice and research closer together.

Canadian nurses tend to look east to the United
Kingdom as well as south to the United States, in
part especially since the introduction of a national
health scheme in Canada. In 1953 the University of
Edinburgh and the Royal College of Nursing accepted
a grant from Boots the Chemists to establish a
research fellowship in nursing in the University of
Edinburgh; and in 1956 the Nursing Studies Unit was
established, prior to the development of the Department of Nursing in the University of Edinburgh
(Simpson, 1971). The Nursing Research Unit was
established in 1971, with Lisbeth Hockey as Director. It was and still is funded primarily by the
Scottish Home and Health Department, in partnership
with the University. Its terms of reference are: to
undertake research into nursing problems within the
health service; to develop appropriate research
tools; to encourage research-mindedness among the
Scottish nursing profession; to teach nurses research methods; and to collect and disseminate
information nationally and internationally (Simpson,
1981, p. 24). This Unit has become a key international centre which attracts researchers from many
countries for varying periods of time.

A nursing research unit was established in 1977
at Chelsea College, University of London, as an
integral part of the Department of Nursing (Cox,
1979). Three multidisciplinary teams, each led by
an experienced researcher and including at least one
nurse with in-depth experience in the problem area,
have developed. A statistician is a member of the
unit staff. The initial focus of this unit was on

problems in nursing education, but has subsequently expanded. It is the only unit which began concurrently with the educational program (Simpson, 1981, p. 25).

In 1979 a third nursing research unit in the United Kingdom was opened at Northwick Park Hospital, funded and developed by the Department of Health and Social Security in association with the Medical Research Council research centre. It is a practice unit headed by a nurse researcher, Rosemary Crowe. The first research project was on pressure sores, a very practical problem both in terms of care and costs (Simpson, 1981, p. 25).

In Canada there has been a variety of clinical nursing research developments. From 1968 to 1970 Margaret Allemang of the School of Nursing, University of Toronto, developed a project to implement, assess and refine a decentralised system of nursing to facilitate patient-centred care in one ward of the Sunnybrook Medical Centre (Allemang, 1971). Within little more than a decade a number of nursing research programs have been developed in clinical settings. Most, but not all, of these programs developed as a joint project of a university faculty of nursing and the nursing department of a major teaching hospital or health centre.

Moyra Allen, a nursing faculty member and a National Health Senior Scientist, developed a centre for nursing research in the School of Nursing, McGill University, in 1974, with funding from Health and Welfare Canada. The first priority of this unit was to demonstrate nursing at a community level including nursing services providing health care for families. A model of nursing was developed to serve as a basis for a number of research projects which described the experiences in nursing and related the practice of nursing to the health outcomes for clients (Allen, 1981). Clinical facilities, known as Health Workshops, were developed by the unit and other clinical settings were used for specific research projects but no satellite unit appears to have been developed within an existing clinical setting. The next clinically oriented nursing research program was developed in Ontario when, from 1980 to 1982, the Sunnybrook-University of Toronto Nursing Project was developed in a major teaching hospital as a joint project (Cahoon, 1981).

Although nursing research in community health services is beginning to develop in the United States, it has not progressed as quickly as that in university faculties of nursing and hospital settings. Also, one must be careful to distinguish between research units and nursing research units. Nurses in community health agencies in Canada have been involved in nursing research for more than half a century but few positions for continuing research in nursing have developed in community settings and for several reasons. Very large community health agencies are beginning to establish research units but these have tended to be primarily statistical and epidemiological in the nature of projects undertaken and few of them have employed nurses on a continuing basis. Most of the community health nurses who have become researchers are employed in university faculties of nursing. There have been few role models for nursing research in provincial or federal departments of health or voluntary health agencies. The practice in community health when a nurse researcher is needed for a particular study has been to second one for a limited time.

Of the various patterns of joint approaches to developing clinical nursing research that have emerged, two dominant patterns emerge. In the first of these a university faculty of nursing and the department of nursing in a major health facility launch a joint project for nursing research within the clinical setting. In the second pattern, a department of nursing in a major health care facility establishes a nursing research unit on an independent basis although some type of cross-appointments to a university faculty of nursing have usually been made for the director and sometimes for some of the other researchers.

The Rationale for Nursing Research in Clinical Settings

Nursing research has been defined as 'systematic inquiry into the problems encountered in nursing practice and into the modalities of patient care, such as support and comfort, prevention of trauma, promotion of recovery, health education, health appraisal and coordination of health care' (Gortner, 1975, p. 193). Nursing research differs from research in nursing in which nursing education, nursing manpower, career patterns, utilisation, costs and the profession itself are studied (Folta, 1968; Notter, 1968).

Nursing research in clinical settings is practice-oriented research, the type of research that should produce beneficial outcomes in terms of the nursing care of patients/clients and their families, groups and communities. Practice research has real potential for convincing patients/clients

and their families, their physicians, other health
care professionals, administrators and governmental
representatives that nursing makes a difference.
Chains and clusters of related studies can be
done in major problem areas in clinical settings and
can be expected to produce more definitive results
than the scattered studies that have been characteristic of the majority of previous research. The
results of independent, isolated studies done by
different researchers in various clinical settings
do not produce cumulative effects, in contrast to
studies that are planned to fit together. Researchers in the related sciences tend to spend years
investigating closely related problems, yet this
type of approach is well suited to nursing research
in clinical settings.

In the Second International Seminar on Nursing
Research, Brotherston argued for the development of
'research mindedness' in all nurses as the basic
move in the development of nursing research. He
said, 'Whereas the ability and opportunity to carry
out research must be limited to a minority in any
profession, an urgent and understanding sense of the
need for research should be a part of the mental
equipment of *every* member of any profession worthy
of the name' (Brotherston, 1960, p. 24). Intermittent investigations in a clinical setting do not
provide the experiential learning that is conducive
to the development of such 'research-mindedness'.

Research is implicit in the roles of all
nurses, whether it is specified in their job descriptions or not. All nurses are exposed to an
increasing amount of research being done in clinical
settings by other health care professionals, chap-
lains, behavioural scientists and even educators,
who are using patients/clients and their families as
research subjects. For example, all nurses have
roles related to the protection of the rights of
patients and families who are the subjects of
research irrespective of who is sponsoring or
conducting it. Although research committees in
institutions and in clinical settings must review
research protocols before research is begun, the
nurses on the care units are those who may observe
questionable ethical practices. They need to know
to whom such practices should be reported.

All nurses have roles relative to the support
of research, especially in the provision of support
to patients/clients and families who are the subjects of studies. They have interpretative roles in
explaining the procedures prior to and during an
investigation. They also have supportive roles in

relation to the activities of researchers. These roles include protection from the unnecessary loss of data and protection against the introduction of sources of bias.

All nurses have roles in the identification of practice problems which should be investigated, roles that are complementary to those of the researchers. Practitioners and researchers must become partners. Other roles are learned by some nurses during practice studies, for example, in some investigations staff nurses may serve as research assistants during data collection and even analysis, whereas clinical nurse specialists may serve as co-investigators.

A major proportion of the important nursing literature is appearing in the form of research reports. All nurses need to become discriminating consumers of research results so that they can make valid judgements about the readiness of results for application in practice.

Many nurses at the staff level in clinical settings have had little basic preparation for these research roles. Further, it is in clinical settings that nurses gain the experiential learning about research that supplements classroom learning.

Clinical settings are the natural fields for the provision of care: general and special institutions, community health services, industry, a variety of health centres and, in nursing, the homes of patients/clients and their families. Research done in any of these clinical settings is research done in the real world of health care rather than in a laboratory or in highly controlled experimental settings. In some very large clinical settings some wards may be more 'controlled' than others for a particular investigation but essentially practice research is done in natural care settings.

The future of the nursing profession is dependent upon research investigation of its practices, rather than of its membership, as 'a means of achieving the kind of caring that is not simple sentiment, but a kind of caring that includes deliberative, scientifically selected action' (Ellis, 1970, p. 444). The ultimate purpose is improvement of patient care. Practice research in nursing is research that can only be done *by* and *with* nurses.

STRATEGIES FOR NURSING RESEARCH IN CLINICAL SETTINGS

Within a clinical facility a nursing research unit can be established in the department of nursing or

in the research department of that facility.
Several of the existing nursing research units in
Canada have been developed within a nursing department, with varying degrees of relationship to that
facility's research department, where one exists.
There can be little doubt that this is the simplest
route at the present time. The structuring of
nursing research within the overall research department of a major clinical setting is probably an
ultimate goal, but that may be difficult or even
impossible to achieve unless attractive sources of
nursing research funds are available from which
there could be some perceived benefit accrued for
the research department as a whole. This strategy
should not be considered unless the nurse researchers and associates can be considered true peers of
those in the other units of the research department.
Without post-doctoral preparation, several years of
experience, and a distinguished track record of
previous research, nurse researchers could be
considered to be in a very subordinate position to
other researchers within such clinical research
departments.

There are various ways in which a nurse researcher can be appointed to develop a nursing
research unit. The most common way is through an
appointment from a university faculty of nursing to
the clinical setting. Such an appointment may be
made from the existing faculty or by recruitment to
the faculty from outside. Appointment of an existing faculty member may shorten the developmental
period of establishing the research unit since the
current interest of an experienced nurse researcher
can be built upon, probably within a few months.
This type of appointment provides for potential for
some time release for other faculty members to
become involved in the studies themselves. The
recruitment of a nurse researcher to a faculty
position for this purpose is additive and does not
entail potential to free up time for other faculty
members. In this type of appointment the developmental period is likely to be longer in that a new
person has to become acquainted with the clinical
area and the research resources of the university.
Yet the new appointee may bring added expertise, new
ideas and relatively few preconceptions. Such
advantages must be weighed against the fact that
such an appointment may carry a message to the
existing faculty that they have not measured up,
which can arouse resistance and become a risk to
morale. Also, it is sometimes difficult to recruit
a nurse researcher who can build upon what has

already been done, as the tendency is for the new appointee to start from her/his research base rather than the collective base evolved by the faculty. Development of independent nursing research units is difficult. Some research positions associated with non-integrated units have been open for very long periods of time, during which time the interest of staff may wane. Very few experienced nurse researchers are likely to seek such positions unless a cross-appointment to a university faculty is assured. This non-integrated approach is possible only for very large health care agencies, and is dependent upon being able to recruit nurse researchers who have depth of knowledge of nursing in the type of health care being given, a broad knowledge of clinical research methodology, substantial research experience and, as emphasised below, on having adequate resources.

SOME MAJOR RESOURCES

The development of nursing research in any clinical setting requires a variety of resources which include personnel, supplies and services, space, funding and time. Some of the resources may already exist while others have to be acquired.

Personnel

One of the most critical resources is a core group of nurses with convictions about the need for nursing research for practice. Ideally, there should be support for nursing research from influential practitioners at all levels, and all administrative staff. Yet in reality, the nurse researchers themselves often have to develop that type of resource.

In many of the nursing research units in existence in Canada development began with the appointment of a single nurse researcher. This practice is likely to continue for some time because of the shortage of nurse researchers and a shortage of funds for such personnel. Such appointments are critical to the development of research, including 'research-mindedness'. The need for well-qualified, experienced researchers cannot be overemphasised. For example, it is unrealistic to appoint a principal nurse researcher to develop a nursing research program in a clinical setting on completion of a master's degree in nursing, despite the fact that a large share of the previous nursing research has been done by nurses with master's level preparation. In fact, some of the most productive researchers have continued to do excellent studies from that beginning base but it must be recognised that most have had formal research training and advanced study of nursing as a discipline well beyond that level and have acquired a much greater breadth and depth of experience. The qualifications and experience of nurse researchers should be as comparable as possible to those of researchers in other fields in the clinical setting. It is usually a better decision to delay such appointments until an able candidate is available.

While availability is a major factor in such an appointment, the pool of nurse researchers in Canada is very small. In a 1976 survey to find out how many nurses were actively engaged in research in nursing, results indicated that 130 were involved in some form of research activity by self-report (Storch, Hazlett & Stinson, 1977). Of these, however, it was estimated that approximately 50 could be classified as a nurse researcher, and only six of them were involved on a full-time basis. In a later study done by the Manitoba Association of Registered Nurses and the University of Manitoba School of Nursing of active nurse researchers in Canada, 213 were identified (Scherer, Cameron, Ramsay, Vogt & Farrell, 1982). The difference is explained in large part by variation in the operational definitions of nurse researcher. In 1980 there were 81 nurses in Canada with an earned doctoral degree, and by 1982 this number had risen to 124. Also, whereas there were 72 enrolled in a doctoral program in 1980, by 1982 there were 121. '[Of the 124 nurses] with an earned doctoral degree, 84 per cent were employed in nursing and related health fields; 73 per cent ... in universities and 11 per cent ... in health care agencies' (Stinson, Larsen & MacPhail, 1984).

Even in relatively small scale nursing research units a principal nurse researcher should have research associates and/or research assistants available to her/him, to become involved in studies and to work with practitioners in the development of research problems. Assistance from statisticians and computer programmers is needed intermittently and if these resources are not internally available in the clinical setting, some external arrangements must be made. Secretarial assistance is also essential.

Supplies and Services
The supplies and services vary with the types of
investigations being done but there are always
requirements for paper, photocopying, reprints,
reference books and, usually, computer services.
Tape recorders and audio tapes and in some centres
video equipment have been used in training data
collectors as well as in collecting data. A pager
for each of the research staff is important if the
clinical setting is large and they are likely to be
coming and going from wards and clinics.

Space
The location of a nursing research unit is important
in fostering the climate for research. If it is
relatively invisible to the nursing staff and/or in
a 'low status' area, they are unlikely to be convinced of its importance. Preferably the unit
should be located within the special facilities
designated for the agency's overall research endeavors, where it will have the potential of gaining the
prestige it deserves.

At least one office for the nurse research-
er(s), a secretary's office, and a workroom are the
minimum required. A conference room is a definite
asset. As research staff increases there must be
potential for additional offices, located close
together.

Funding
Nursing research development requires adequate
funding assured over a period of several years. It
is doubtful whether a nursing research unit can ever
become self-supporting, because there are usually
gaps between the end of one grant and the beginning
of another. Little, if any, research today can be
done without funding. Most provincial governments
in Canada appear not to be ready to include the
costs of nursing research in budgets for nursing
services and in this author's opinion they are
unlikely to provide even minimal funding until and
unless nursing research becomes more visible and
demonstrates its effectiveness and efficiency.

Although some clinical settings have developed
their own research funding program from which small
grants have been allocated for specific nursing
studies, this source is likely to provide little
more than 'seed' money. There are a number of
granting agencies to which applications may be made
but there is always a considerable period between

application and review; further, the proportion of
proposals that receive funding may be as low as 20
per cent. Currently, there appears to be less
funding available in Canada for practice studies
than for studies focused on nursing education and
manpower.

Time
Although less tangible than many of the other
resources, time is most important. Will it be
possible to release practitioners to assist in
nursing research without stealing time from patient
care? Are practitioners ready to accept that nurse
researchers have to have time to read what others
have done, talk with colleagues, and think before
making decisions that are critical in research
planning, as well as write proposals, protocols and
reports? While practitioners develop quick decision-making and carry out relatively visible activities, the work of researchers tends to be much less
visible and appears to take a long time to demonstrate results. Such differences can become a
source of conflict if practitioners and researchers
do not understand each other.

THE FORCE FIELD FOR DEVELOPMENT

The development of nursing research in a clinical
setting is a process of planned change. Lewin's
three steps for planning change (1952) were used in
the six-year project to investigate the feasibility
of increasing nursing research activities through a
regional effort, by the Western Interstate Conference on Higher Education in Nursing (Krueger, Nelson
& Wolanin, 1978), and have also been used in development at the institutional level. These three
steps are:

1. An unfreezing, by making a previously stable
    state amenable to change. This can be accom-
    plished by one of several strategies: provi-
    sional involvement; direct confrontation;
    acceptance of ambivalence; and/or creation of a
    vacuum.

2. Moving to a new level, based on the multitude
    of factors unique to each case. This step is
    subdivided into four steps by Lippitt, Watson,
    & Westley (1966) in which the individual
    establishes relationships, clarifies problems,

examines alternative solutions and goals, and transforms intentions into actual change efforts.

3. Freezing at a new level or attainment of a new equilibrium...

(Krueger et al., 1978, p. 302).

Some of the forces in any clinical setting facilitate research development while other forces inhibit it. In the development of a nursing research unit, nurses at all levels have to create a climate for research that builds upon the supportive factors and reduces the restraining factors. While lowering an inhibitor may be more effective than strengthening a facilitator, in such a marked change, the supportive forces have to be developed.

Some nursing research units have grown from staff research interest groups which began during lunch hours. In a hospital in Toronto, at the first of such meetings, a nurse researcher was invited to present a brief report of a study and its implications for practice, followed by open discussion of potential trials of applications. If sufficient interest is aroused through these approaches, more time may be made available for different activities such as problem identification, reviews of what has already been done in previous studies on a specific problem, and what could be done. Although such research groups tend to be small they identify those nurses with real interest and enthusiasm for research activities and they facilitate sharing of ideas and information among them.

Nursing research committees have developed out of such interest groups in some settings and have sometimes been developed on the basis of some type of framework for research development. The objectives may be very limited in the beginning but may extend over time to include encouragement of research for the provision of optimal care, to plans for the provision of journal clubs, seminars and other learning opportunities, and even to the co-ordination of some of the research-related activities.

In some committees nursing research protocols are reviewed and recommendations are made to approve or not approve specific projects. This process may include reviewing all research proposals or only those submitted from outside individuals and agencies. In the review process it is important that the nursing research committee members be aware of other research that is being done at a particular time in that agency in order to protect patients from being 'over-researched' and to protect staff from excessive demands for special data collection. In some clinical settings the research committee may develop a roster of consultants for nursing research. Some of the individuals may be in other departments and others may have to be sought from a university or outside facility.

The library facilities for nursing research are limited in many clinical settings and a research committee may develop files of nursing research reports, funding agencies, and make recommendations for acquisitions. There are many free newsletters available from various sources which contain information about activities in other centres that would be of interest to practitioners and senior administrators.

For example, the Committee on Clinical Nursing Research of the Hospital of the University of Pennsylvania, Philadelphia, produces a nursing research newsletter within the hospital and university to disseminate information about nursing research activities and to recognise nurses involved in studies and work groups (Fuhs & Moore, 1981). This committee has developed an exciting program of activities that is stimulating research involvement. Such a committee may also promote the publication of research reports by staff members and encourage them to make presentations at professional meetings.

In terms of investigation, the committee or a group of its members might become involved in replication of a study of interest in several units within the clinical setting. Other groups might become involved in the application of research results in one or more units. A set of guidelines along these lines was developed for the WICHEN Project (Krueger et al., 1978, p. 364) which is a very practical aid to assessing the generalisability and utility of nursing research findings.

Krueger has proposed a structured approach to planning and using clinical nursing research findings in practice (1977, 1978). She has identified nursing administrators as facilitators of change (1978) and has also pointed out the roles of nurses in middle management in nursing research (1979). With administrative leadership an active research committee may take on responsibility for a large part of the co-ordination of the nursing research activities within the Department of Nursing.

In most instances it is wise to establish an advisory or steering committee prior to planning for the development of a nursing research unit and the introduction of one or more nurse researchers. If there are other research committees in the clinical setting there should be cross-representation. If the nursing research program is to be part of the facility's overall research program, there should be clear agreement on who is responsible for providing what supplies and services, etc. In such circumstances it is also usually advisable to begin with one nursing research theme or problem area which is of crucial concern to a number of the related research units within the facility.

Padilla proposed that similarities between the research process, the nursing process, problem-solving and evaluation can be used in introducing the nurse researcher to the staff in the clinical setting (1979). Some researchers may think that this approach is an over-simplification of the research process, but it could be useful as an interpretive strategy during the transitional phase.

Even in planned change some resistance is functional for the preservation of a degree of stability, yet there is always resistance that is unwarranted. In any development attention has to be focused on reducing the restraining forces. Some of the resistance may arise from within the nursing department and some of it may come from without.

In the nursing department if there are insufficient numbers of staff and/or too few staff with advanced expertise, resistance may emerge if staff perceive research development simply as an additional responsibility without additional resources being introduced. It may be difficult for staff to support nursing research unless they can be convinced that it is only through careful investigation that service needs can truly be substantiated. Also, and to their credit, practitioners usually have to be convinced that patient care needs will always override research requirements.

If there is instability of staff in the clinical setting, morale may be threatened, and an attitude of let someone else do it may develop. Attention needs to be focused on such problems and staff must be helped to understand that research results may help them in achieving more stability and better morale.

Resistance may arise from medical researchers and their colleagues in the related sciences if they feel threatened about losing complete control of research in the clinical setting. In at least some Canadian clinical settings the control of research has been placed in the hands of medical staff to the point where a physician has to sponsor a nursing study. And in some instances a physician has insisted on co-investigator status and on co-author status in the report, whether or not he/she had been substantively involved. On the other hand, several early nursing research developments in Canada were supported by interested physicians who collaborated with the nurses in their studies. Fidler pointed out that support from physicians rather than resistance had been encountered (1952). Some physicians are still true colleagues and respect the research that nurses have done and are doing. Probably the greatest difficulty has been that of a communications problem; some nursing studies have not been understood by medical scientists, and/or that the quality of some of the previous nursing research has not been a very good advertisement. Reducing the communications gap may be difficult if the physicians avoid explanations. When challenged about quality this author has replied that she can find as poor examples in their field as in her own for that period in time, and also she has given physicians literature on exemplary nursing research.

Disapproval of patient/client and family participation by one or more physicians can do considerable harm to the inclusiveness and reliability of the patient sample in a practice study. Involvement of visible, supportive physicians in nursing research planning and activities will probably do more to reduce resistance than any other single factor.

A low-keyed approach to the introduction of a nursing research unit may arouse less resistance than too much visible attention. Development takes time and dissatisfaction may arise if unrealistically high expectations have been set. Although some of the outcomes are tangible, some progress toward meeting the following criteria should be evident at the end of a three-year period:

1. Chains and clusters of problems in a clinical area have been investigated in a manner that will enable research results to have greater utility than was likely to occur from small, independent and unrelated investigations.

2. Involvement of clinical nurses and other health professionals interested in clinical problems in nursing should be increasing.

3. There should be increase in funded research although this may depend upon the general

problem area and the availability of grants for this kind of research in the field of enquiry.

4. There should be improvement in the quality of the research climate of the setting.

5. There should be increase in the use of research results in clinical practice.

6. There should be increase in the research knowledge of staff and their support for nursing research.

SUMMARY

The origins of nursing research were in clinical settings. The real focus for nursing research, the practice of nursing, was identified more than a century ago. There is now a revival of nursing research in clinical settings in Canada, the United States and the United Kingdom.

Practice research has the potential for convincing colleagues and consumers that nursing makes a difference. Chains and clusters of related studies in clinical settings can produce cumulative results whereas independent, isolated investigations cannot. The development of research mindedness in all professional nurses requires opportunities for experiential learning in clinical settings. Practice research requires partnership between practitioners and researchers. Practice research in nursing is research that can only be done *by* and *with* nurses.

Two major strategies for the development of nursing research units in clinical settings have emerged: a joint project of a department of nursing of a major teaching hospital and a university faculty of nursing, and an independent unit in a clinical setting. As yet, the pool of qualified and experienced nurse researchers is small. One of the most critical resources in the clinical setting is a core group of nurses with convictions about the need for nursing research for practice. Funding is essential, and over a period of several years.

The development of a beginning climate for research should precede the development of a nursing research unit. There are many activities through which nursing staff can influence the research climate and continue to learn about research.

If nurses do not rise to the challenge of research of their own practices, they will find decisions being made on the basis of research done by others -- who may not ask the relevant questions nor be able to interpret the responses. The future of the nursing profession is dependent upon its own research of its practices.

NOTE

Editor's Note: 'American' here refers to the U.S.

REFERENCES

Abraham, G.E. (1968). Promoting nursing research in an organized nursing service. *American Journal of Nursing, 68*, 818-821.

Allemang, M.M. (1971). A project to implement, assess and refine a decentralized system of nursing to facilitáte patient-centered care. Toronto: School of Nursing, University of Toronto (mimeographed).

Allen, M. (1981). A model of nursing: A plan for research and development. In Proceedings of the International Conference *"Research - A Base for the Future?"* (pp. 315-330) Edinburgh: Department of Nursing Studies, University of Edinburgh.

Brotherston, J.H.F. (1960). Research-mindedness and the health professions. In International Council of Nurses and Florence Nightingale Foundation, *Learning to investigate nursing problems* (p. 24).

Bunge, H.L. (1958). The Institute of Research and Service in Nursing Education, Teachers College, Columbia University. *Nursing Research, 7*, 113-115.

Cahoon, M.C. (1981). The interdependence of nursing research and practice. In Proceedings of the International Conference, *"Research - A Base for the Future?"* (pp. 340-345). Edinburgh: Department of Nursing Studies, University of Edinburgh.

Carnegie, M.E. (1978). Quo vadis? *Nursing Research, 27*, 277-278.

Cox, C. (1979). The nursing education research unit: The early days. *Nursing Times, 75*, 747-749.

Decary, M. Souer (1956). L'hopital Notre-Dame de Montreal aborde la recherche en nursing. *Bull. Infirm. Cath. Can., 23*, 1-4.

Ellis, R. (1970). Values and vicissitudes of the scientist nurse. *Nursing Research, 19*, 440-445.

Folta, J.R. (1968). Conference on the nature of science and nursing: Perspectives of an applied scientist. *Nursing Research, 17*, 502-505.

Fuhs, M.F., & Moore, K. (1981). Research program development in a tertiary care setting. *Nursing Research, 30*, 24-27.

Gortner, S.R. (1975). Research for a practice profession. *Nursing Research, 24*, 193-197.

Hanson, R.L. (1971). Research in nursing service. *Nursing Outlook, 19*, 520-523.

Harmer, B. (1932). School for Graduate Nurses, McGill University. In *Methods and problems of medical education*, 21st series. New York: Rockefeller Foundation.

Kopf, E.W. (1961). Florence Nightingale as a statistician. *Quarterly Publication, American Statistical Association*, NS 13, 388, 404.

Krueger, J.C. (1977). Utilizing clinical nursing research findings in practice: A structured approach. *Communicating Nursing Research, 9*, 381-384.

Krueger, J.C. (1978). Utilization of nursing research: The planning process. *Journal of Nursing Administration, 8*, 6-9.

Krueger, J.C. (1978). Nursing administrator's roles in research: The WICHE program. *Nursing Administration Quarterly*, 2:27-31, Summer.

Krueger, J.C. (1979). Nursing research and the middle manager. In A. Marriner (ed.), *Current perspectives in nursing management* (pp. 142-155). St. Louis: C.V. Mosby.

Krueger, J.C., Nelson, A.H.N., & Wolanin, M.O. (1978). *Nursing research: Development, collaboration and utilization.* Germantown, MD: Aspen Systems Corp.

Lewin, K. (1951). *Field theory in social science.* New York: Harper & Brothers.

Lippit, R. (1966). The process of utilization of social research to improve social practice. In A.B. Shostak (ed.), *Sociology in action: Case studies in social problems and directed social change.* Homewood IL: Dorsey Press.

Nightingale, F. (1859). *Notes on nursing.* London: Harrison & Sons.

Nightingale, F. (1963). *Notes on hospitals* (3rd ed.). London: Longman, Roberts & Green.

Notter, L.E. (1968). The nature of science and nursing (editorial). *Nursing Research, 17,* 483.

Padilla, G.V. (1979, January). Incorporating research in a service setting. *Journal of Nursing Administration, IX(1),* 44-49.

Scherer, K., Cameron, C., Ramsay, J., Vogt, C., & Farrell, P. (1981). Methodological considerations in the construction of national data bases: Identification of and access to Canadian nurse educators and researchers in a target population. In Proceedings of International Conference, *Research - A Base for the Future?* (pp. 229-236). Edinburgh: Department of Nursing Studies, University of Edinburgh.

Schlotfeldt, R. (1975). Research in nursing and research training for nurses. *Nursing Research, 24,* 180.

Scott, D.W., Oberst, M.T., & Dropkin, M.J. (1980). A stress-coping model. *Advances in Nursing Science, 3,* 9-23.

Simpson, M. (1971). Research in nursing: The first step. *International Nursing Review, 18,* 231-247.

Simpson, M. (1981). Issues in nursing research. In L. Hockey (ed.), *Current issues in nursing* (pp. 19-32). Edinburgh: Churchill Livingstone.

Stinson, S.M. (1986). Nursing research in Canada. In S.M. Stinson & J.C. Kerr (eds.), *International issues in nursing research*. London: Croom Helm.

Stinson, S.M., Larsen, J., & MacPhail, J. (in press). *Canadian nursing doctoral statistics: 1982 update*. Ottawa: Canadian Nurses Association.

Storch, J., Hazlett, C.B., & Stinson, S.M. (1979). Nurses involved in research. *Dimensions in Health Service, 56,* 34-35.

Werley, H.H. (1962). Promoting the research dimension in the practice of nursing through the establishment and development of a department of nursing in an institute of research. *Military Medicine, 127,* 219-231.

Werley, H.H. (1972). This I believe ... about clinical nursing research. *Nursing Outlook, 20,* 718-722.

Woodham-Smith, C. (1950). *Florence Nightingale.* London: Constable.

Chapter Twelve

SCIENTIFIC REPORTING IN NURSING

M. Elizabeth Carnegie

Considering that the first report of a scientific investigation was published, probably by Aristotle, in the 4th Century, B.C., nurses as members of a young profession or discipline are relative newcomers to the publishing scene. Florence Nightingale's monumental study of health and hospitalisation in the British Army in the mid-nineteenth century initiated the recognition of publication by nurses. Further, her many other well-known writings based on her scientific investigations brought about significant changes in health care, not only in the British Empire, but throughout the world. Nightingale, recognised worldwide as the first nurse researcher, 'possessed in abundance the qualities of the good researcher: insatiable curiosity, command of her subject, familiarity with methods of inquiry, a good background in statistics, and ability to document and abstract' (Palmer, 1977, p. 88).

HISTORY OF NURSING PUBLICATIONS

In the United States, writing by nurses for publication started in 1888 in Buffalo, New York, with the appearance of the *Trained Nurse*, which, in 1893, absorbed another magazine, *Hospital Review*, which became the *Trained Nurse and Hospital Review* afterwards. It was not, however, until the turn of the century that nursing established its own official magazine, the *American Journal of Nursing* -- owned, edited, and controlled by nurses. The first issue appeared on October 1 of that year and continues to be the professional journal of the American Nurses' Association. From 1900 to 1950, there were about eight nursing magazines exclusive of bulletins of state and district nurses' associations and nursing school alumni organisations.

Although published by a university and not intended to duplicate the official nursing journals, reference must be made to another publication. Between 1928 and 1943, Teachers College of Columbia University in New York published *Nursing Education Bulletin* twice a year. This was a publication devoted to study and experimentation. As an experimental project, the *Bulletin* carried reports of studies by students and faculty.

In the 1950s, five new magazine titles appeared, including *Nursing Research*. In the 1960s, several more were added, some scholarly with reports on research in nursing, but with a brief lifetime, e.g. *Nursing Science*. In the 1970s, a magazine explosion was experienced and more have appeared in the 1980s, making a total of more than 60 today in the United States alone; however, not all are controlled by nurses.

Since their inception, national nursing associations around the world have published for their members official magazines, bulletins, newsletters, and the like. In addition, for nearly 30 years nurses in all member countries of the International Council of Nurses have been served by the *International Nursing Review*, a bimonthly journal. Current nursing publications from all countries -- books, monographs, articles, reports, conference and colloquium proceedings, directories, and doctoral dissertations -- are listed regularly in the *International Nursing Index*, published quarterly by the American Journal of Nursing Company in New York.

EVOLUTION OF RESEARCH REPORTING

In reviewing reports of early nursing studies, there is virtually nothing in the sparse nursing literature that refers to scientific reports by nurses in the United States before 1900. However, through the efforts of nursing leaders, the movement of nursing into the university had begun in 1899 with the offering of a course in hospital economics for nurses at Teachers College, Columbia University, New York. This was the first step toward university recognition of the nurse's need for higher education.

Before the magazine, *Nursing Research*, was born in 1952, the vast majority of articles by nurses based on research -- not complete or scholarly reports -- were published in the *American Journal of Nursing*. In its first decade of existence, the *Journal* published five articles based on studies by nurses: a survey of visiting nurse societies in the country, then numbering 53, highlighting progress, operations, and future plans (Fulmer, 1902); a report of 500 cases of pneumonia cared for by visiting nurses, along with statistics (Hitchcock, 1902); a study of morbidity and mortality due to dirty milk (Goler, 1904); economic use of surgical supplies, e.g. gloves and gauze (MacDonald, 1906); and a description of a nurse's invention of an appliance for surgical beds, which she had patented by the U.S. Patent Office (Richards, 1906).

The first editorial on research was carried in the *American Journal of Nursing* in 1906. This editorial was based on the awarding of cash prizes to senior students at Lakeside Hospital in Cleveland, Ohio, for essays on nursing care. The purpose of the contest was 'to encourage and stimulate the powers of observation, to develop the ability to write intelligently on the knowledge gained, for the express purpose of gleaning information that may be of value to the nursing profession and to mankind.' Topics for these essays were selected by the Training School Committee and the one selected that year was 'The Alleviation of the Discomforts Following Anaesthesia' (Research work done by nurses, 1906).

The results of Nutting's survey of nursing education, conducted in 1906, was published by the U.S. Commission of Education under the title, 'The Education and Professional Position of Nurses' (Nutting, 1907). This was probably the earliest, most important study of nursing education in the United States by a nurse. Other significant works by nurses based on research in this first decade were Nutting and Dock's two-volume *History of Nursing* (1907) and Waters' report on visiting nursing in the nation, based on a survey sponsored by the American Nurses' Association (Waters, 1909). It has been said that this historical report, which showed variations in policies and practices, led to or hastened the founding of the National Organisation for Public Health Nursing, a forerunner of the National League for Nursing. Research reports were also included in the *Trained Nurse and Hospital Review, Public Health Nursing*, and many publications in the form of books and monographs of the then three major national nursing organisations -- the American Nurses' Association, the National

League of Nursing Education, and the National Organisation for Public Health Nursing -- were based on research.

In the twenties, we saw members of other disciplines entering the nursing research arena, perhaps for economic reasons rather than to enhance nursing research. For example, the first study reported in the nursing literature was conducted by a Ph.D. for the New York Academy of Medicine on the nursing situation in hospitals (Lewinski-Corwin, 1922). This study uncovered the hospital practice of permitting more orders to be written for nursing procedures than could be executed by the available staff.

Of the 259 published articles identified as having been based on nursing research between 1900 and 1952, the vast majority dealt with registered nurses -- their functions, activities, economics, and general welfare as private duty nurses and as nurses in hospitals and public health agencies. In nursing education, most of the articles focused on curriculum; nursing service articles focused on procedures; the few clinical articles were mostly in the area of maternal-child nursing. Sixty percent of the authors were nurses; others included educators, statisticians, a few industrial engineers, and social scientists. Most of the studies were instigated and published by the major national nursing organisations.

Not only was there a growing interest in research on the part of organised nursing in the first half of the century, but as schools of nursing moved into universities, more nurse scholars began to affirm their belief that they too must engage in research as one of the major functions of the university; also recognised was the need to disseminate their findings through publication. Therefore it was logical that the Association of Collegiate Schools of Nursing (ACSN) develop and sponsor a publication devoted to informing the nursing profession and others about the results of scientific studies in nursing and to stimulate research. In 1950, the Association of Collegiate Schools of Nursing, with the approval of the other national nursing organisations and the offer of financial assistance from the American Nurses' Association, spearheaded the movement for a magazine devoted exclusively to reporting research in nursing. ACSN made the first financial contribution and became the sponsoring organisation for the new magazine, *Nursing Research*, which published its first issue in June, 1952. Launched by the

American Journal of Nursing Company, it continues to be published by the Journal Company which provides editorial and managerial services and absorbs all costs in excess of subscription revenue.

Before the advent of *Nursing Research*, nurses had come to realise that scientific study of nursing problems was mandatory in order to improve their practice and hence improve the quality of patient care. In that period, we saw nursing organisations, individually and collectively, involved in research on the welfare of the nurse in the areas of nursing education, hospital nursing service, and public health nursing, and the literature reflects their research efforts.

Until the seventies, *Nursing Research* was the only journal in the United States devoted exclusively to reporting research, but other countries had begun comparable publications in the sixties. In England, it was the *International Journal of Nursing Studies*; in Japan, the *Japanese Journal of Nursing Research*; and in Canada, *Nursing Papers*. *Nursing Papers*, a medium for assessing problems, posing questions, and describing ideas and plans of action by those concerned with nursing research, is a publication of the School of Nursing at McGill University in Montreal, and serves as the official organ of the Canadian Association of University Schools of Nursing.

The late seventies produced four more scholarly journals -- one in England and three in the United States. The *Journal of Advanced Nursing*, published in England, made its debut in 1976 followed in 1978 by *Research in Nursing and Health*, a John Wiley and Sons (New York) publication, and *Advances in Nursing Science*, published by Aspen Systems Corporation in Maryland. In 1979, the *Western Journal of Nursing Research*, published by Phillips-Allen in California, made its appearance. As with scientific journals in other disciplines, these research journals are all refereed -- a system that helps a magazine maintain standards and foster quality control of scientific communications.

THE REFEREE SYSTEM

Regardless of the discipline, scholarly journals are refereed by a panel of judges with expertise in various types of research -- basic and applied, in content areas, and in methodology. The review process is done anonymously and the peer reviewers, or referees, follow certain guidelines -- general and specific:

General

1. The content is consistent with the purpose of the journal.

2. The article makes a contribution toward the advancement of scientific knowledge or research methodology.

3. The content is organised and presented clearly in a manner consistent with the usual standards and format of a scientific journal.

Specific

1. The problem has been stated clearly.

2. The review of the literature shows how the study is based on previous thinking in the field or how it is intended to extend it.

3. The relationship of studies of the problem, or closely related problems by other investigators, is shown or it is placed in the context of relevant works done previously in the problem area.

4. Key terms are defined clearly.

5. Assumptions and limitations are stated.

6. The research design is appropriate for the problem and is described clearly.

7. The data collection method is appropriate and adequately explained.

8. If human subjects are involved, in an experimental investigation especially, the investigator gives evidence of how their rights have been protected.

9. The sample is representative to the extent that the results can be generalised.

10. The instruments, or tools for the data collection, are appropriate for the study and are described adequately.

11. Under findings and results, data are discussed.

12. Appropriate statistical tests are used in analysing the data and are reported.

13. Conclusions are drawn on the basis of the data and reflect positive and/or negative results.

14. References are adequate for the subject (Carnegie, 1975).

According to a recent survey, of the 25 responding editors of nursing journals in the United States, 23 reported that their journals were refereed (Clayton & Boyle, 1981). Another survey included journals in other countries. Of these 22 respondents, 12 -- located in Canada, India, Switzerland, England, New Zealand, and Zambia -- indicated that their journals were refereed, but most of the editors added such qualifying terms as on occasion, whenever necessary, and varies (Mirin, 1981).

A refereed journal has been defined in many ways. In general, it is agreed that 'A refereed journal is one which utilises a system of pre-publication review by three or more readers who judge the merit of manuscripts according to the criteria established by the journal' (Clayton & Boyle, 1981, p. 534).

Zuckerman and Merton (1971, p. 100), both eminent sociologists and researchers, point out that 'The system of monitoring scientific work before it enters into the archives of science means that much of the time scientists can build upon the work of others with a degree of warranted confidence. It is in this sense that the structure of authority in science, in which the referee system occupies a central place, provides an institutional basis for the comparative reliability and cumulation of knowledge.'

SHIFTING EMPHASIS AND INVESTIGATORS

In comparing the kinds of research published by nurses in the first half of the 20th Century with that from the mid-century on, we see a shift in research emphasis and investigators. Emphasis has shifted from research in such areas as teaching, administration, curriculum, recruitment, careers, and the practitioner herself to clinical studies with the objective of improving the quality of patient care through the research process. Research in nursing addresses the human and behavioural questions that arise in the treatment of disease, prevention of illness and maintenance of health. Much of this emphasis on research in patient care and evaluation of it may be attributed to more institutions -- educational and service -- promoting and supporting nursing faculty and/or staff in their research efforts; the establishment of research centers at universities, clinical facilities, and those operated by nursing organisations; and the increasing number of research councils, forums, seminars, and conferences.

Research conferences and the like are occurring on all levels: international, national, state/provincial, and local -- international, e.g. the Workgroup of European Nurse Researchers; national, e.g. the National Research Conferences in Canada, the Royal College of Nursing of the United Kingdom Research Society, and the American Nurses' Association Council of Nurse Researchers; regional, e.g. the Western Council on Higher Education for Nursing of the Western Interstate Commission for Higher Education and the Eastern Conference on Nursing Research; state/provincial, e.g. those sponsored by these nursing associations; and local, e.g. the many chapters of Sigma Theta Tau, the national honor society of nursing in the United States and Puerto Rico, usually sponsored jointly with a university. Such conferences give nurses an opportunity to share their research findings with their peers and disseminate that knowledge orally and through the published proceedings.

In recent years, we've seen a shift from research in nursing conducted largely by members of other disciplines, especially the social scientists, to that conducted almost exclusively by nurses themselves. More and more nurses are principal investigators of research studies, with members of other disciplines serving as co-investigators. A large part of this has been due to the fact that more nurses are being prepared at the doctoral level to conduct scientific investigations. We have come from one nurse with an earned doctorate in the late 20's (Edith Bryan), to about 150 by the end of the fifties, to slightly over 500 by the end of the sixties, to 1,019 in 1973, including 55 nurses employed in 18 countries[1] other than the United States (American Nurses' Foundation, 1973), to 2,348 in the United States alone seven years later (American Nurses'

Association, 1980). It should be pointed out that
the numbers reported here are based on those nurses
with earned doctorates who responded to a mail
questionnaire and that the 1980 ANA survey was not
international in scope. So the total number of
nurses in the world with doctoral degrees is really
unknown.

A BRIGHT FUTURE

For years, research findings reported in the
literature by nurses was almost nonexistent.
Today, *with* the number of nurses prepared on the
graduate level to conduct research, with the
growing number of doctoral programs in nursing
(more than 20 in the United States to-date and a
developing one in Canada), with the increasing
number of outlets for nurses to disseminate their
research findings, with expanding opportunities for
nurses to present their studies at conferences and
symposiums where they can be critiqued objectively
by peers, with more institutions encouraging nurses
to experiment and supporting them -- financially
and otherwise -- in their research efforts, with
more and more health care institutions employing
nurses as directors of research, with the establishment of research centers in nursing, and with
nurses' own desire to develop theories and find
answers to nursing problems through the research
process, nursing research has finally come into its
own.
    Nurses are searching for new facts by collect-
ing data in a rigourously controlled situation for
the purpose of predicting, explaining phenomena,
and finding answers to nursing problems. They are
taking the final step in the research process --
communicating the results through the printed word
to members of the profession, scholars and others
for the purpose of advancing knowledge. DeTornyay
(1977, p. 10) predicts that in the future nursing
research findings will be shared with scientists in
other disciplines to a much greater extent.
'Knowledge gained from research,' she says, 'is not
knowledge owned by any one group, and nursing
research must be shared with others in places where
they will have access to it.' DeTornyay speaks of
the future, but nurses are already publishing in
scholarly journals of other disciplines, e.g.
medicine, law, sociology, psychology, anthropology,
education, hospital administration, public administration, and business. Also articles based on

research written by nurses for the lay public are appearing in such respected general magazines as *Good Housekeeping,* the *Ladies Home Journal,* and the *Saturday Evening Post.*

The future looks bright for nurses to be able to share their research through many publishing outlets -- international media; federal and state/provincial agencies; national, regional, state/provincial, and local nursing organisations; foundations; universities; health service agencies; learned societies; book publishing houses; and scholarly journals of other disciplines.

Today, research and the reporting of it by nurses, is being given high priority by the nursing profession and is beginning to be recognised by other professions and the general public as a necessary, scholarly activity. Through their published works based on research, nurses are showing that good nursing care prevents hospitalisation in many cases, shortens hospital confinement and is cost effective.

NOTES

1. Australia - 1, Canada - 28, Chile - 1, Colombia - 1, Egypt - 1, India - 3, Ireland - 1, Israel - 2, Italy - 1, Japan - 1, Korea - 1, Peru - 1, Poland - 1, South Africa - 1, Switzerland - 2, Thailand - 2, Uganda - 1, and the United Kingdom - 6 (England - 5 and Scotland - 1). Seventeen of these 55 nurses with earned doctorates are from universities in eight countries other than the United States: Canada, England, Germany, Japan, Poland, Scotland, South Africa, and Switzerland.

REFERENCES

American Nurses' Association (1980). *Directory of nurses with doctoral degrees.* Kansas City, Mo: Author.

American Nurses' Foundation (1973). *International directory of nurses with doctoral degrees.* New York: Author.

Carnegie, M.E. (1975). The referee system (editorial). *Nursing Research, 24,* 243.

Clayton, B.C., & Boyle, K. (1981). The refereed journal: Prestige in professional publication. *Nursing Outlook, 29*, 531-534.

deTornyay, R. (1977). Nursing research -- the road ahead. *Nursing Research, 26*, 404-407.

Fulmer, H. (1902). History of visiting nurse work in America. *American Journal of Nursing, 2*, 411.

Goler, G.W. (1904). Nurses' work in milk stations. *American Journal of Nursing, 4*, 419.

Hitchcock, J.E. (1902). Five hundred cases of pneumonia. *American Journal of Nursing, 3*, 169.

Lewinski-Corwin, E.H. (1922). The hospital nursing situation. *American Journal of Nursing, 22*, 603.

MacDonald, M.V. (1906). Economy in the use of surgical supplies. *American Journal of Nursing, 6*, 676.

Mirin, S.K. (1981). *The nurses' guide to writing for publication.* Wakefield, MA: Nursing Resources.

Nutting, M.A., & Dock, L.L. (1907). *A history of nursing.* New York: G.P. Putnam's and Sons.

Palmer, I.S. (1977). Florence Nightingale: Reformer, reactionary, researcher. *Nursing Research, 26*, 84-84.

Research work done by nurses (Editorial). (1906). *American Journal of Nursing, 6*, 350-351.

Richards, E.H. (1906). Miss E.H. Richard's invention. *American Journal of Nursing, 6*, 232.

Waters, Y. (1909). *Visiting nurses in the United States.* New York: Charities Publications Committee.

Zuckerman, H., & Merton, R.K. (1971). Patterns of evaluation in science: Institutionalism, structure, and function of the referee system. *Minerva (London), 9*, 99-100.

Chapter Thirteen

**NURSING RESEARCH IN THE UNITED KINGDOM: THE STATE
OF THE ART**

Lisbeth Hockey

INTRODUCTION

This chapter is intended to give an overview of
nursing research in the United Kingdom; it does not
claim to be exhaustive in this rapidly expanding
subject area. Because of the diversity of interpretation of nursing research, definitions used in
this contribution are given below:

Research: an attempt to expand the body of
available knowledge through a process of
systematic scientific enquiry.

Nursing: those activities and duties which
constitute the appropriate and predominant
work of professionally qualified nurses. It
is recognised that such work varies between
countries and also changes over time within
any one country. In the U.K. such work includes not only nursing practice in the clinical setting, but also preventive care, such as
health education, nursing education and nursing administration at all levels of management.

Nursing Research: an attempt to extend the
available body of knowledge relevant to nursing work through a process of systematic
scientific enquiry.

Art of Nursing Research: research, being a
process of identifiable stages, requires a
modus operandi for each stage; the art refers
to these modi operandi.

State of the Art: state has a temporal conno-
tation and must be considered against the
background of the past and the prospects for
the future.

How one views the past and what one perceives
and desires for the future is, to a large extent,

subjective and influenced by one's personal position. The subjectivity of this chapter is readily acknowledged.

Framework
Several possibilities for the structuring of this chapter presented themselves; the selection of the framework was made after considerable thought and was eventually guided by an attempt to provide information which could be subjected to international comparisons and which could be condensed within the limitations of one chapter. The literature on the development of nursing research, from whatever country it originates, seems to agree broadly on seven basic requirements and these provide the framework. They are:
1. Individual academic curiosity.
2. Research education.
3. Research activity.
4. Appropriate research climate.
5. Research finance.
6. Dissemination of research related information.
7. Research utilisation.

The first part of the chapter presents a personal view on the position of nursing research in Britain in relation to the seven requirements. In the second part, the focus is on research activity in the three main spheres of nursing, that is nursing education, nursing practice and nursing administration. The chapter concludes with a subjective appraisal of past performance and an equally subjective glimpse into the future.

Neither individual research reports nor names of researchers are singled out and the chapter, therefore, lacks a conventional reference list or bibliography; the number of references which would have qualified for inclusion in this widely ranging chapter militated against it. Several nurse researchers could have been mentioned as having made a significant contribution to the development and the advance of the art of nursing research; it would have been easy to overlook others.

The mention of names in conjunction with specific posts such as directors of research units makes little sense at a time of rapid change; indeed, contact may be delayed rather than aided if individuals have moved elsewhere. The decision was made, therefore, to provide a list of the main sources of information about all aspects of nursing research, which should be reasonably enduring.

PART I. THE STATE OF THE ART IN RELATION TO THE
SEVEN REQUIREMENTS FOR THE DEVELOPMENT OF NURSING
RESEARCH

1. Individual Academic Curiosity

There can be little doubt that the opportunity for
academic nursing education has contributed to a
questioning attitude of nursing students although
evidence for a causal relationship between education and academic curiosity has not yet been established. It is normal practice for undergraduate
students to pursue individual problem solving and
to look critically at the activities they are
taught. Questioning is encouraged and academic
teaching staff are aware of their responsibility to
provide their students with research based information and to present relevant alternatives. It is
not intended to imply that *all* academic teaching
staff actually discharge their responsibilities in
this way or that teaching staff in the conventional
non-academic nursing schools have no research
awareness; such a deduction would be far from the
truth. Teachers are also individuals and their own
academic curiosity and teaching style are individually determined. However, an academic setting
lends itself more readily to an imaginative educational approach. In the U.K. academic settings are
increasing rapidly and, therefore, the number of
nurses who have the opportunity of an academic
education alongside their professional preparation
to become licensed practitioners is also rising.
Currently, there is somewhat of a plateau because
of the economic constraints, but this applies to
all nurse learners not merely to undergraduate
students. In the U.K., academic education for
nurses is not restricted to universities; courses
are also provided by some technical colleges and
polytechnics. In those cases degrees are awarded
by the National Council for Academic Awards (NCAA).
The curricula offered in courses approved by this
body, which are nationally standardised, make
provision for project work and the need for research based teaching is given due emphasis. The
newly constituted National Bodies responsible for
nursing, midwifery and health visiting also have
declared the importance of research awareness in
education. Thus, in relation to individual academic curiosity, newly qualified nurses, whether
graduates or not, have normally been exposed to and
encouraged in questioning and reasoning. Unfortunately, such individual curiosity tends to be

stifled later and it seems to require a great deal of determination to retain it.

2. Research Education

There appears to be agreement that research education must be provided at three levels simultaneously if the nursing profession is to be truly research based. In the U.K. notable advance has been made on all three fronts and the current position can be summarised as follows:

(a) Research Appreciation. This is considered as the basic level of research education which ought to be offered to all members of the nursing profession. Its purpose is not only to encourage individual academic curiosity as described above, but also to enable nurses to read research reports with a measure of understanding. In many health service establishments up and down the country brief courses of a few days to around two weeks are held; in addition, the national bodies responsible for nursing education are encouraging and approving clinical nurse study courses on research appreciation. As Keighley (1984) reports, two new courses have been approved very recently, one in Nottingham, England, the other at the Royal Marsden Cancer Hospital in London. The Nursing Studies Research Unit at Edinburgh (Scotland) University, the University of Manchester (England) and the Royal College of Nursing in London as well as in Wales, Northern Ireland and Scotland have been offering courses of one to two weeks' duration for many years. Most post-basic professional nursing courses have a research appreciation component, largely based on the curriculum pioneered by the Joint Board of Clinical Nursing Studies, the national body which was responsible for post-basic clinical nursing education before the new national structure for all professional education became operational in 1983.

(b) Research Methodology. In contrast to research appreciation, courses in research methodology aim to give nurses the basic tools for research. It is reasonable to assume that all nursing education in the tertiary sector includes research methodology. Such education refers not only to undergraduate programmes but also to post-graduate ones at master's and doctoral levels. Although, doctoral preparation in the U.K. does not have a set course programme, students are normally encouraged to undertake appropriate methodology courses either within departments of nursing or in other university departments. Seminars and other post-graduate activities afford the opportunity for the acquisition of some further knowledge on research methodology.

(c) Research Involvement as Assistants. The difference between this method of research education and the other two, outlined above, is the learning by doing. Within the last five years, the opportunities for nurses to be attached to research projects have increased markedly. The establishment of Nursing Research Units has been a significant factor in the development of nursing research in the U.K. Since 1971, when the first such Unit was established within the Department of Nursing at the University of Edinburgh, five major Units came into being. All of them have a nurse as Director and all of them offer posts for nurses as research assistants.

3. Research Activity
As stated in the introduction to this chapter, the state of the art relating to research activity is the concern of Part II. In the context of this summary, suffice it to say that the number of research projects undertaken by nurses is rising rapidly. Most of those projects form either part or the whole of post-graduate education, leading to either a master's or a PhD. degree. A survey of nurse researchers conducted by the Nursing Studies Research Unit in Edinburgh, indicated that about 60% of nurse researchers in 1980 undertook their research for a research degree (Laing and Johnson, 1982).

4. Appropriate Research Climate
Nursing research cannot flourish unless administrators create a conducive atmosphere for its growth. As alluded to above, the individual academic curiosity with which many newly qualified nurses enter their professional career tends to be stifled in an agency where routine and convention rule the day and where the inspired hunches of individual nurses tend to get either ignored or even ridiculed. Such instances are, fortunately, getting less common but

they are still encountered. The U.K. is currently
in a stage of transition, not only in relation to
new legislation in nursing education (Nurses,
Midwives and Health Visitors Act 1979), but also in
the structure of the National Health Service
(Health Services Act 1980). Transition tends to be
linked with uncertainty and personal uncertainty of
senior nurses does not readily lead to the initia-
tion of research which generates further uncertainty. Uncertain people prefer to tread on safe
ground which is more likely to be found in convention than in investigation. However, since the
reorganisation of the National Health Service in
the wake of the new legislation in 1980, new posts
were created for nurses to take responsibility for
research. The idea of such posts may be seen as a
great potential for research development; unfortunately, many incumbents have found themselves in
positions of extreme frustration, either because
the expectations of what can be achieved are unrealistic or because they feel themselves inadequately prepared in research. Attempts to alleviate the
situation on both fronts are being made. Courses
in top management include facilitation and utilisation of research as well as the elements of research methodology. Research interest groups have
been established in many parts of the U.K. and
attempt among other objectives to provide peer
group support for relatively lonely research workers. The Royal College of Nursing, through its
Society of Nursing Research, is currently discussing more effective means of helping such nurses.
Access to clinical research areas has been difficult to achieve in some health care agencies.
There are encouraging signs of improvement, mainly
through the greater participation of nurses on
ethics committees. The provision of finance for
the development of nursing research can be considered as part of an appropriate research climate and
it is certainly necessary for nursing administrators to face up to this responsibility. Because
finance is a crucial factor it is discussed more
specifically below.

5. Research Finance
In the U.K. research finance is available from
three main sources. These are:
(a) Government research funds.
(b) National Health Service funds at local levels.
(c) Private Trusts and Foundations.

In addition, finance for nursing research may be provided by research councils, such as the Medical and Social Science Research Councils and some funds may be available from universities and polytechnics.

In the U.K., by far the most significant funding source for nursing research is the Department of Health and Social Security (DHHS), which is the Government Health Department for England and Wales and its Scottish counterpart, the Scottish Home and Health Department (SHHD). The survey of nurse researchers in 1980 indicated that approximately 40 per cent of all research was financed from government research funds, followed by approximately 35 per cent from National Health Service local sources. At a seminar on nursing research in 1982 at DHHS, it was stated that DHHS funds for nursing research during 1982-3 amounted to approximately one million pounds sterling. Government research funds are made available in a variety of ways. In the first instance, three nursing research units are financed in this way, two by DHHS and one by SHHD; these are referred to in greater detail below. Through the medium of the Nursing Research Liaison Groups (NRLG) within DHHS and the Chief Scientist Office (CSO) within SHHD, the government may use research funds to finance specific projects, either in response to grant application or by commission. Both Government Health Departments, that is DHHS and SHHD, also award Research Training Fellowships to nurses, thereby contributing to the preparation of nurse researchers. Some government monies may be made available to universities and polytechnics for nursing research.

As far as the NHS funds at local level are concerned, nurses must compete alongside the other health professions. History seems to suggest that nurses have been relatively slow in claiming these funds and that their medical colleagues have been more successful. As more nurses acquire the skills of grantsmanship, one may look forward with some realism to a larger slice of the locally available financial cake for nursing research.

Private trusts and foundations have some of their assets ear-marked for research and are, therefore, a helpful additional resource. In the U.K., the Nuffield Provincial Hospitals Trust, the King Edward's Hospital Fund, the Leverhulme Trust and the Edwina Mountbatten Trust featured most prominently as funding sources for nursing research.

To the category of private monies should be added a large number of voluntary agencies and industries which may give money for specific projects which fall within their sphere of interest. The number of nurses who have successfully attracted funds from such sources has shown an encouraging increase in recent years.

6. Dissemination of Research Related Information

The rapid increase of nursing research in all fields of nursing inevitably poses problems of dissemination of findings and other relevant information, especially research in progress. At the Seminar referred to above, the difficulty of dissemination was identified as a major problem area. In the U.K. constant efforts are being made to improve the situation, the most important among them being effected through the co-operation of librarians. A unique information service dealing with U.K. nursing research was established by and within DHHS in 1975. This information service, described by Stodulsku and Stafford (1982) led to a quarterly abstracting journal, *Nursing Research Abstracts*. These are derived from the *Index of Nursing Research*, also established in 1975, as an expansion of a comprehensive information system which had been developed over the preceding ten years by nursing officers in the Research Section of the Nursing Division at DHHS. The *Index* is based on a thesaurus of nursing terms and is capable of conversion to computerised retrieval. The part-time librarians responsible for the maintenance of the *Index* respond willingly to enquiries by nurses and spare no effort in helping nurses to use information sources effectively.

The other main centre for research related information is the Royal College of Nursing Library. It publishes a monthly Nursing Bibliography which is freely distributed; it includes nursing literature of all kinds, not merely research literature. Again, the librarians respond readily to requests for help and advice.

In Scotland, the Health Services Library, maintained by the Manpower Services Division, holds a large stock of literature, including research reports. It also compiles specialised bibliographies on specific subjects, for example, pressure sores, ward design, nursing equipment, nursing research.

In order to facilitate the dissemination of research normally only available in thesis form and restricted to university libraries, the Royal College of Nursing Research Series was initiated in 1973 with financial backing from DHHS Research and Development funds. The series represents edited versions of the original theses, making the work more readily available to and intelligible for nurses outside the academic system.

Nurse researchers and librarians continue to work together in order to facilitate the dissemination of information even further. The survey of nurse researchers (*op.cit.*) suggested that nurse researchers themselves do not find the communication and dissemination of research adequate and pin-point lack of education and lack of availability as the major weaknesses.

The appointment of nursing research liaison officers at regional levels in some parts of England and the newly created posts of Research Nurses within the National Health Service have the potential of improving the communication and dissemination channels.

7. Research Utilisation

The ultimate objective of research effort is the utilisation of findings which is clearly linked with all the other requirements for the development of research outlined above. Utilisation is not synonymous with implementation, a term which tends to be used too loosely. Utilisation includes the deliberate rejection of a research report either because of its poor quality or because of its irrelevance. No use can be made of it if it is not read or not understood. Utilisation also includes the critical assessment of a specific research method with a view to using it in another setting. On the whole, the U.K. nursing profession has not demonstrated much headway in the utilisation of research in any way.

Utilisation of research should also include the benefits which could be derived from knowledge which is not necessarily intended to have a direct application for the nursing service. It would be regrettable if the value of fundamental research were to be underestimated or even negated.

Lack of generalisability of research findings tends to be the main reason for lack of implementation. Most nursing research in the U.K. has been of a small scale, undertaken by single-handed researchers; therefore, results could not be generalised and their potential as change agents was not recognised. Because most nursing research is

undertaken by post-graduate students working for a
research degree, replication of research undertaken
by others is not popular; thus, many excellent
studies are lost to the profession. Surveillance
of the international nursing literature suggests
that this problem is not unique to the U.K. It is
an extremely important international problem to
which the nursing profession should address its
attention.

PART II. RESEARCH ACTIVITY

A chapter on the state of the art relating to
research activity in nursing can be expected to
have an evaluative approach; the reader who has
such an expectation will be disappointed. Moreover, no individual research efforts are being
singled out for special consideration; consideration was given to a selective evaluative survey
but this self-imposed task was found to be not only
prohibitive but also invidious. The selection of
material would be too subjective and guided by
personal interest and limited competence to be of
value to a diverse readership. The decision was,
therefore, made to present a factual cursory overview of the main research endeavour in the U.K., to
comment on structure and thrust rather than on
methodological details.
  It seems reasonable to begin this overview
with the main centres of research activity in the
U.K., the established research units and other
centres with a concentration of research activity.
The three units, mentioned earlier as being funded
by the government health departments are:
i.   Nursing Research Unit, Department of Nursing
     Studies, University of Edinburgh, established
     in 1971 and financed by the Scottish Home and
     Health Department.
ii. Nursing Education Research Unit, Department of
     Nursing, University of London (Chelsea Col-
     lege), established in 1977 and financed by the
     Department of Health and Social Security.
iii. Nursing Practice Research Unit, Northwick Park
     Hospital and Clinical Research Centre, estab-
     lished in 1979 and financed by the Department
     of Health and Social Security.
Other Nursing Research Units, established within
the last decade are variously placed and financed:
o   The Nursing Research Unit within the Royal
     Marsden Cancer Hospital is financed by the
     Board of Governors of that Hospital.

o   The Nursing Studies Unit within the Faculty of
      Medicine at the University of Nottingham is
      financed by Regional Health Authority research
      funds.
o   The Daphne Heald Research and Development Unit
      within the Royal College of Nursing was estab-
      lished through voluntary fund raising and
      needs to attract further finance for its
      research work.
o   A Nursing Policies Study Centre is currently
      being established within the University of
      Warwick with funding from the King Edward's
      Hospital Fund for London.

All units have responsibility for research
activity as well as the collection and dissemination of information; some, for example the units in
Edinburgh and Nottingham, provide some structured
educational opportunities for nurses outside the
university system. All units have a Director who
is a qualified nurse with additional research
training and experience. Additional research
workers are employed at two levels: project leaders
and assistants. Project leaders may not be nurses;
it depends on the specific expertise and experience
which is required. Research assistants are normally nurses, as these posts afford valuable opportunities for research training.

As far as the thrust of the research activity
is concerned, the names of the units indicate their
main interest in most cases. Thus, the Nursing
Education Research Unit is developing as a centre
for research into education - currently midwifery
and clinical nursing education; the Nursing Practice Research Unit has its focus on nursing practice, currently pressure sores. The Unit within
the Royal Marsden Hospital concerns itself with
different aspects of cancer nursing, such as pain
control, the prevention of chemotherapy-induced
alopecia, care of mastectomy patients, etc.

The first of these Units, in Edinburgh, at-
tempted to identify those areas for research which
the Scottish nursing profession seemed to be concerned about. After its early major descriptive
study which was published as a guide for novice
researchers, it developed a programme of research
into different aspects of communicating in nursing.
A change of Director in 1983 is likely to change
its theme. The two Units most recently established, *viz.* in the University of Nottingham and
the Royal College of Nursing, are pursuing nursing
practice research problems, such as stoma care.

The distinctive feature of research units versus other research centres is their financial structure. Funding is provided for the Unit and includes provision for core research staff, secretarial support staff and equipment. It is in the growth of such units that the U.K. seems to have made significant progress and, as far as one is able to ascertain, there are extremely few such units specifically for nursing research in other parts of the world.

Nurse researchers are also employed as directors, project leaders or research assistants in other related Units, such as the Health Services Research Unit in the University of Durham.

Centres of concentrated research effort tend to be in universities with departments of nursing, notably the University of Manchester. This Department together with the Nursing Research Unit in the Department of Nursing Studies in Edinburgh are also the two Collaborating Centres in the U.K., exploring the "Nursing Process" as part of the WHO (Europe) Medium Term Programme in Nursing and Midwifery. All university departments of nursing have teaching staff with a research commitment and all have academic responsibility for post-graduate research students. Some polytechnics also have a research focus, notably the Polytechnic of the South Bank in London and the Sheffield City Polytechnic. In Scotland, the College of Technology in Dundee has a well developed Department of Nursing with a significant research involvement.

It is difficult to find an agreed method by which to categorise nursing research, a kind of typology. For the purpose of this chapter the broad headings of nursing education, nursing practice and nursing administration are used.

Nursing Education
In the U.K. nursing education was the first area to be tackled by nurse researchers and a considerable effort continues to be made in order to explore the many aspects of nursing education. They include studies of recruitment, wastage or attrition, adaptation to being learners, teaching methods, especially the relationship of theory to practice, the acquisition of clinical nursing skills and many others. The new structure of nursing education in the U.K., implemented in 1983, affords opportunity for new approaches to nursing education research. Greater centralisation ought to facilitate access to clinical learning areas and to colleges of

nursing and midwifery. As far as the current state of the art is concerned, it is fair to claim a fair level of sophistication in research designs and methods, with a healthy balance between quantitative and qualitative approaches. Instruments for the measurement of clinical competencies are being designed and tested. The national examination system is being subjected to increasing exposure to test its validity and reliability. National data bases are being established and increasingly experimental research in controlled settings is being conducted.

Nursing Practice

Nursing practice research includes all of nursing and, therefore, the current state of the art is extremely amorphous. As background to the present scene, mention must be made of the Royal College of Nursing Project which, over a period of six years in the '70s, pursued various aspects of the quality of nursing care. The project resulted in a series of twelve monographs. They include studies on dressing techniques, feeding of unconscious patients, pre-operative fasting, bowel care in hospital, patient anxiety, etc. The project deserves special mention because it provided 12 nurses with some research skills and the topics studied paved the way for further nursing practice research. Two of the studies were experimental in design which, a mere ten years ago, constituted a breakthrough in British nursing research. The design and evaluation of nursing equipment also forms part of nursing practice research and in the U.K. nurses are actively involved in the preparation of research based specifications of various articles of nursing equipment; it is, however, still a largely unexplored research area.

The care of incontinent patients including possibilities for the prevention of incontinence, the prevention and nursing treatment of pressure sores, including incidence and prevalence studies and various aspects of communication in nursing, are topics which have been and are being most consistently explored by nurse researchers. More recently, patient views have been included in evaluative nursing practice studies. Nurses in the U.K. join the chorus of nurses the world over in clamouring for instruments to measure the quality of care; they look for solutions to researchers who, in turn, expect practising nurses and, especially their teachers and administrators, to state

criteria of high quality care which might be incorporated in a measuring device. The goal is still
beyond reach. What is being achieved in the U.K.,
is a much greater awareness of the need for a sound
scientific base and a well defined conceptual and
theoretical framework for practice research.
Nurses are beginning to ask more incisive questions
and the design of their studies fits more comfort-
ably into serious research arenas, deserving the
approval of the most skeptic scientist. It is no
longer necessary nor possible for nurse researchers
to have any special consideration where the competition for funds is concerned. Therefore, their
research proposals have to conform to the general
rules of utmost scientific rigour. It is gratifying that on that basis nurse researchers have been
awarded sizeable research grants. It must be
stated, however, that such successes are still confined to a minority of nurses and some funds,
potentially available for nursing research, pass
nurses by only because of inadequately prepared
proposals.

Some nursing practice research lends itself
particularly well to a multi-disciplinary approach:
the care of the elderly, the dying, antenatal care,
infant feeding, etc., represent just a few examples
where nurses have worked well with other disciplines. Whereas even just a few years ago nurses
working within an inter-disciplinary team would
have been merely data collectors, they are now able
to make their own professional contribution to the
research; as already indicated, in some instances
nurse researchers have held and are holding leadership positions in multi-disciplinary teams. In
this context it is probably relevant to note that
most nurse graduates in the U.K. and particularly
those with a post-graduate qualification also have
a specific academic education in one of the sciences underlying nursing, for example psychology,
sociology or biological sciences. With the development of more degree courses *in* nursing, this
situation is likely to change and the change may
alter the type of nursing practice research being
undertaken. The survey of nurse researchers in
1980 (*op.cit.*) indicated that nursing practice
research was undertaken by about 40 per cent of the
respondents. This figure is not totally reliable
as many nurses found it difficult to place their
research into one of the three categories of practice, education or administration; the analysis of
the answers provided under *other* showed that much
research crosses these artificial boundaries.

Nursing Administration

The organisational framework in which nursing takes place cannot be ignored in any nursing research, even if it does not always have priority consideration. The organisational framework includes the policies which control nursing practice, it determines the number and the mix of staff, the number of learners in the clinical situation, the lines of communication between the ever increasing number of care providers, etc. Studies in the field of organisational structures have tended to have a sociological or an operational research orientation, but nurses have been involved in both types. A specific contribution by nurses has been the development of nursing dependency measures to help in the calculation of nursing workload and appropriate staffing. Studies of nursing records, the use of computers in ward management, research into nurses' sickness rates and absenteeism also fall within this category.

The current emphasis in this type of research in the U.K. seems to be on attempts to calculate staffing needs. Most of the many formulae developed for this purpose have been based on nursing dependency measured in a variety of ways. The use of individualised nursing care plans for the estimation of workload was introduced by a Canadian nurse in one hospital in Scotland (Grant, 1979). Replication of this small study would be timely. The new Nursing Policy Research Unit at the University of Warwick can be expected to be fully operational by the time of publication of this volume. It is bound to introduce a specific slant into the study of policy formulation and its work should provide badly needed knowledge in this important area of nursing. An encouraging innovation within the administrative structure is the appointment in a few authorities of well qualified nurses with clinical and research responsibilities.

PART III.   CONCLUSIONS

The Past and the Future

One's impression of past achievements and one's futuristic ideas are bound to be totally subjective and coloured by one's own experiences.

However, by any standard, a rapid impressive growth of nursing research in all areas within the last decade must be acknowledged. A development which does not fall into one of the three broad areas outlined above, but which must not be discounted, is historical research. At least five doctoral theses within the last five years have pursued historical work and a group of nurse historians has been established within the framework of the Royal College of Nursing.

It is gratifying that more research centres have been established in spite of the economic recession, that research training fellowships have, with the exception of one brief break in England and Wales, been continued and that nurse researchers have been able to attract funds for individual projects from a variety of sources. Probably the most marked progress has been made in the number of nurses who have received research training and have been awarded PhD degrees. This progress would be even more gratifying if those nurse researchers were able and willing to continue to explore the subject areas of their interest, thereby deepening the knowledge within them. Unfortunately very few, if any, nurses with research competence seem to be thus employed. The trend is for such nurses to work in institutions of higher and further education, mainly in universities, where research nearly always takes second place to teaching and other responsibilities. The other posts which qualified nurse researchers occupy are, understandably and appropriately, administrators of nursing research units. As stated in Part II, the directors of all such units in the U.K. are nurses. As directors of nursing research or health care research units such nurses must apply themselves to the wider sphere of work undertaken within the unit, leaving them little time for any personal research in a narrow subject area.

In spite of the increase of research activity it is, as yet, not possible to find many examples of research constituting a change agent. In fact, it seems to have made little impact on nursing and, only too often, tradition and convention still have the upper hand. Significant progress might be made with the introduction of more research based teaching material and journals; there are promising signs in this direction but there is still a very long way to go.

What has been achieved is a greater research awareness and those nurses who wish to pursue their awareness are likely to find research based literature which may help them either by deepending [*sic*] the understanding of their activity and its underlying concepts. Some research reports might suggest different methods of care but, almost invariably, such suggestions are not conclusive. A personal and somewhat cynical view of research literature is that it seems to be used to the greatest advantage by nurse researchers in the compilation of their bibliographies. Nurse researchers are in the danger of setting themselves apart, creating yet another of the many elite groups within our profession.

It is this view of the past which, whilst freely recognising achievements, is tinged with some pessimism and disappointment and must colour the final futuristic glimpse - fears as well as hopes for nursing research in the U.K. First, the fears: Nurse researchers may merely perpetuate their own species without due concern for the future of the profession as a whole. If research cannot be demonstrated as having made even the slightest difference to nursing, it may become increasingly difficult to make claims for monies or time for it.

Unless a change of attitude towards research is adopted by the senior members of the nursing profession, that is administrators and teachers, two harmful consequences are likely. In the first place, intelligent young people who have been encouraged already within their basic school education to undertake projects, and to enjoy problem solving, will not readily enter a profession where these exciting possibilities do not exist. Secondly, the gap between theory and practice and the gap between the academic community and the nursing profession outside academia are likely to increase. The chances of changing any part of nursing because of research are likely to decrease rather than increase and the declared aim of making nursing a research based profession will remain a cliche rather than become a reality.

Finally, the hopes: Nursing, in the U.K., now has unprecedented opportunities for radical change. The increase of nurse scientists and competent nurse researchers has the potential of introducing into all aspects of nursing a truly scientific perspective and dimension. The hope that this potential may be exploited must surely be shared by all who have a genuine interest in the advance of the nursing profession. Nursing research must become an integral part of everyday thinking of nursing professionals.

It is reasonable to hope that any research based education in nursing schools of every kind will be applied in the clinical learning situations. If and when nursing education in the U.K. becomes truly unified in terms of theoretical and clinical education, such transference of a research approach will be easier to effect. Further, in terms of the organisational aspects, the inclusion of nurses on all ethics committees must be achieved for the preservation of the professional integrity of nursing research.

The most sincere hope of all is that all members of the nursing profession may become eager to engage in productive thinking and may learn to enjoy the pleasures of it. Such thinking would be the most effective means of bringing together the two essential attributes of any true profession, namely academic and professional. Antagonism and mistrust which some practitioners have in relation to academics and the patronising, if not scathing, attitude which some academics have in relation to practising nurses must and will give way to mutual understanding and respect. The different personalities, skills, interests and levels of competence which nurses bring to their professional activity must and will be used to the advantage of all workers and harmonised for the benefit of the increasingly complex and challenging health care of patients and clients.

It is also hoped that the encouraging international exchange of views and knowledge will continue. In all countries of the world, health care of the population hinges upon effective nursing - restorative and preventive. In the last decade a great deal has been achieved; in the next one we must see a much greater realism in the expectations of academic researchers and a much greater desire for research based knowledge among all members of the practising nursing profession. A realisation of this hope is the most certain way of allowing research to become a change agent and to achieve the WHO goal for the year 2000 - Health for All - or at least access to its possibility.

NOTES

1. The exceptions are: Survey of Nurse Researchers in 1980 (Laing & Johnson, 1982) because it is used as source for this chapter and the study undertaken by the Canadian nurse (Grant 1979) because she is no longer working in the U.K.

REFERENCES

Grant, N. (1979). *Time to care*. London: Royal College of Nursing.

Health Services Act (1980). Chapter 53. London: HMSO.

Keighley, T. (1984). Prologue for the future. *Nursing Mirror, 158(1)*.

Laing, E., & Johnson, R. (1982). *Survey of nurses associated with research in 1980. Proceedings of the RCN Research Society XIII Annual Conference, Royal College of Nursing*. London.

Nurses, Midwives and Health Visitors Act (1979). Chapter 36. London: HMSO.

Stodulski, A.H., & Stafford, S.M. (1982). Disseminating nursing research information in the U.K.: Nursing research abstracts from the Index of Nursing Research. *International Journal of Nursing Studies, 4*, 231-236.

Material used in the preparation of this chapter:

DHHS Handbook of Research and Development (1981). London: HMSO.

Nursing Research Liaison Group Seminar (1982). *A Development of research in nursing*. Unpublished report by DHHS, obtainable from DHHS under C.N.O. 82(10).

Lelean, S.R. (1980). Research in nursing: An overview of DHHS initiatives in developing research in nursing. *Nursing Times, Occasional Papers, 76* (3&4).

Sources of research related information in the U.K.:

Research Units:

Nursing Studies Research Unit, University of Edinburgh, 12 Buccleuch Place, Edinburgh, EH8 9JT, Scotland.

Nursing Education Research Unit, Chelsea College, University of London, Kings Road, London SW10.

Nursing Practice Research Unit, Northwick Park Hospital and Clinical Research Centre, Northwick Park, Watford Road, Harrow, Middlesex, HA1 3UJ.

Nursing Studies Unit, Department of Medicine, Nottingham University, University Park, Nottingham, NG7 2RD.

Nursing Research Unit, Royal Marsden Hospital, Fulham Road, London, SW3 6JJ.

Daphne Heald Research and Development Unit, Royal College of Nursing, 20 Cavendish Square, London W1M 0AB.

Government Departments:

Principal Nursing Officer (Research), Department of Health and Social Security, Alexander Fleming House, Elephant and Castle, London, SE1 6BY.

Nursing Officer (Research and Manpower), Chief Scientist Office, Scottish Home and Health Department, St. Andrew's House, Edinburgh EH1 3DE, Scotland.

Index of Nursing Research, Department of Health and Social Security, Alexander Fleming House, Elephant and Castle, London SE1 6BY.

Libraries:

Chief Librarian, Royal College of Nursing, 20 Cavendish Square, London, W1M 0AB.

Chief Librarian, King's Fund Centre, 126 Albert Street, London, NW1 7NF.

Chief Librarian, Scottish Health Services Centre, Crewe Road, Edinburgh EH4 2LF, Scotland.

Other main source of information:

United Kingdom Central Council for Nursing, Midwifery and Health Visiting, 23 Portland Place, London, W1N 3AF.

Chapter Fourteen

NURSING RESEARCH IN CANADA

Shirley M. Stinson

In one sense, nursing research in Canada is a topic which spans several centuries, back to the 17th Century when Jeanne Mance and her fellow nurses tried out various ways of improving the care of the sick in what was then Lower Canada. Within the 20th Century, the Canadian Nurses Association's history of its first 60 years (CNA, 1968) stands as testimony not only to specific studies of nurses and nursing during those decades but to important groundwork laid for the development of nursing research in Canada. Many additional factors and events were important in the gestation period but, looking back, it would seem that the 'birth' of Canadian nursing research was in 1971. That was the year that some 375 nurses from across Canada and from all sectors of nursing gathered together in Ottawa at the first national nursing research conference. That was the turning point. Nursing research in Canada was finally, irreversibly, on its way.

A definitive description of the development of nursing research in Canada is yet to be written. As such, a limitation of this chapter is that much of the content is simply that of a first-person account. The author's major objective is to provide nurses internationally with a *'coup d'oeil'*, an overview of some of the major antecedents and current characteristics of nursing research in Canada.

Attention is first directed to key Canadian nursing research sources, then to six major characteristics of nursing research in Canada. Little reference is made to the financing of nursing research as that topic is covered in Kerr's chapter. Lastly, a perspective on the topic is cast in the form of an epilogue. Throughout, a developmental approach is taken, the underlying theme being that nursing research doesn't just 'happen'. It is the result of a number of dynamic, complex factors and forces -- and to some extent. chance.

Literature Sources

Without question, the most outstanding repository of literature relating directly and indirectly to nursing research in Canada is the Canadian Nurses Association's Helen K. Mussallem Library at CNA headquarters in Ottawa. It is the envy of many other national professional nursing associations, and Canadian nurses can be proud of this resource.[1] It contains copies of hundreds of Canadian nursing studies, including masters' theses in nursing and Canadian nurses' doctoral dissertations; reports of research projects funded through major external bodies (such as the National Health and Research Development Program); and studies conducted by provincial nursing associations, health care agencies, and various individuals. Beginning in 1964 with CNA's *Index of Canadian Studies* (CNA, October 1982), such studies have been catalogued by topic, author and title. Still, it must be emphasised that as yet a comprehensive catalogue of all Canadian nursing research does not exist, and there is no one repository which contains a collection of all the major studies.

Reports on completed nursing research projects funded by the National Health Research and Development Program (NHRDP) are available through the National Health Science Library. The dissertations of Canadian nurses completing doctoral degrees in recognised universities in North America are available on loan from those universities through Interlibrary Loan, or can be purchased from University Microfilms in Ann Arbor, Michigan.

In terms of ongoing nursing research, the most significant information base is the Canadian Clearinghouse for Ongoing Research in Nursing (CCORN), developed by Dr. Amy Zelmer at the University of Alberta in 1976. This is a public file computerised system which can be accessed across Canada and which currently contains over 100 entries of nursing research being done within and outside the universities. The current Director of CCORN, Dr. Janice Morse of the University of Alberta Faculty of Nursing, has recently expanded the CCORN data base to include a (bilingual) CAMN database of all completed (since 1963) Canadian nursing masters' theses.

Additionally, those new to Canadian nursing research may find the following sources instructive. They contain detailed information on specific research projects and/or are useful references on the development of nursing research in Canada:

o Proceedings of the national nursing research conferences.
o *Nursing Papers*, a refereed journal aimed at scholarly articles and research reports, published quarterly by McGill University since 1968.
o Simms' inventory (1972) of nursing research studies in Alberta, subsequently updated yearly by the Alberta Association of Registered Nurses.[2]
o Stinson (1977), a description of central issues in nursing research in Canada.
o Zilm, Larose and Stinson (1979), a collection of papers from the Kellogg National Seminar on doctoral preparation for Canadian nurses.
o The Canadian Nurses Association's 'Background Paper', a broad overview of facilitators and barriers in nursing research (CNA, 1981).
o The 'Report of the Medical Research Council's Workgroup on Nursing Research' (1985), the most recent document[3] on national trends, issues and priorities.

METHODOLOGICAL AND CONTENT EMPHASES

Even within the last decade, there have been shifts in emphases in the methodology and content of investigations undertaken by Canadian nurse researchers.

Methodology
As emphasised earlier by this author (in Zilm et al., 1979), 'no other single academic or professional discipline reflects the use of such wide-ranging [research] methodologies as does nursing' (p. 14). Canadian nursing research reflects emphasis on both deductive and inductive approaches. Dr. Moyra Allen, Canada's most illustrious nurse researcher, and Dr. Helen Glass of the University of Manitoba pioneered the application of grounded theory to the investigation of nursing phenomena, starting in the late 60s. Descriptive research predominates but, as papers given at national research conferences in Canada indicate,

experimental and historical approaches are not uncommon. The methods and concepts employed cover the gamut from symbolics to empirics, esthetics, ethics, synnoetics and synoptics.

Geographically, the scope of research projects ranges from local, provincial to national studies and, recently, some international projects.[4] Units of analyses range from microscopic to macroscopic. Evaluation research is on the increase, as are studies involving complex data analyses and computer simulations.

Behavioristic thinking dominated much of Canadian nursing research in the '70s, but the search for reasons and intent (i.e. phenomenological research) is starting to edge out the 'cause and effect' school of thought. Conceptual frameworks are now the norm, many of them holistic in nature. However, in the strict sense, no Canadian nurse researcher has as yet employed holographic theory.

This author's cursory appraisal of some fifty recently completed Canadian nursing research projects indicates increased attention to establishing the validity and reliability of instruments, and a propensity to base research not only on some type of conceptual framework but, increasingly, on some type of *nursing* framework. While many of the projects fall short of being rigorous, the evidence indicates an improvement in the quality of questions and designs compared to a decade ago.

Content

By the late '60s, a shift from studies focused on nursing education to those on nursing service had taken place (Poole and Stinson, 1974, p. 185). By the mid '70s, another shift had begun: toward research on nursing practice. It is beyond the scope of this chapter to detail specific studies, but preliminary materials prepared by members of the Medical Research Council's Working Group on Nursing Research[5] indicate a wide range of content. Some examples of types of content are as follows:

o Patients' perceptions of illness.
o Families' reactions to cancer.
o Comfort measures to reduce tension.
o Developing and testing tools to measure quality of care.
o Continence and confusion in the elderly.
o Nurses' stress in differing environments.
o Developing nursing diagnoses.

o Improving the reliability of measures of patients' nursing care needs.

What constitutes the 'domain' of nursing research is becoming less contentious *within* Canadian nursing. But the nursing profession in Canada has for the most part as yet to convince related health professionals, academics, research policy makers and the public at large that nursing is a professional discipline in its own right, with a research focus that is distinctive. This brings us to the larger question of what is the social significance of nursing research in Canada.

SOCIAL SIGNIFICANCE

The question of the social utility of research is certainly not peculiar to nursing. But, by and large, most Canadians have never heard of 'nursing' research, albeit that the Minister of Health and Welfare, the Honourable Monique Begin, gave recognition to the importance of nursing research in a recent speech delivered in Geneva ('Statement...', May 3, 1983).

Canada spends over six billion dollars a year on nursing services (Stinson, 1983, p. 92). From a research and development standpoint, if it spent even one per cent on nursing research, that would be some 60 million dollars annually. Yet this author estimates that the all-time high spent in any one year was 1.7 million dollars in 1979, and that subsequently less than $700,000 per year has been spent on nursing research. (In some years, the total amount was less than $400,000.) In contrast, the amount spent on medical *qua* medical research by 1984 exceeded 175 million dollars.

Fagin, an American nurse researcher, maintains that 'in aggregate [the U.S. studies she surveyed] provide extremely compelling evidence that nursing research is making significant contributions to the health care of our [U.S.] society despite minimal public and private support' (1982, p. 2). It would appear that both in the United States and Canada there is as yet little societal recognition given to the actual and/or potential significance of nursing research.

It is widely acknowledged that many complex factors determine what is or is not viewed as socially significant in any one culture. Thus, lest Canadian nurses become discouraged at what seems to be lack of substantial recognition of the

societal value of nursing research, one should keep
in mind not only that nursing research is a compar-
atively new development but also the fact that only
recently have women begun to penetrate the political power structure in Canada, much less penetrate
the decision-making on scientific and health research policy matters. The prime exception at the
national level is that from its inception, the
National Health Research and Development Program
has appointed nurse researchers to its policy and
review committees, and at the provincial level, the
Board of the Alberta Foundation for Nursing Research, composed primarily of nurse researchers.
    Nursing research may well *be* socially signifi-
cant in Canada, but what ultimately matters is that
it is also *perceived* to be significant.

NURSING RESEARCH MANPOWER

There is widespread agreement within the profession
that there is a paucity of nurse researchers in
Canada. Of some 215,000 registered nurses in
Canada, only some 11 per cent are qualified at the
baccalaureate level and only one-half per cent hold
a master's degree (Statistics Canada, 1982).
Findings from a national survey sponsored by the
Canadian Nurses Association (Stinson, Larsen and
MacPhail, 1984) indicate that in 1982 Canada had
124 nurses with earned doctoral degrees (less than
15% having a doctoral degree in nursing *per se*),
and 121 nurses currently enrolled in a doctoral
program in Canada (66%) or elsewhere (34%). Admittedly, these numbers constitute a considerable
increase over those reported in the 1980 survey: 82
with an earned doctorate and 71 currently enrolled
(Larsen and Stinson, 1980). But given the denomi-
nator, Canada has relatively few nurses with advanced research training.
    In that it is not empirically sound to argue
that only nurses with a doctoral degree can do
research, Canada's current nursing research manpower potential may be seen by some countries to be
considerable. Yet some 125 nurses with doctorates
and less than 2,000 with master's degrees does not
constitute an adequate nursing research manpower
base when one considers: the total population (over
25 million); the vastness of the country (nearly
four million square miles); the numbers of university nursing (24) and diploma and college nursing
(over 100) programs; the numbers, complexity and
dispersement of hospitals and health units,

government health departments, private clinics, industrial health services; and the fact that, in large part due to the nationwide medicare and hospitalisation coverage introduced in Canada in the mid '50s and supported by federal-provincial funding, Canadians have come to expect the best in health care.

There are few full-time nurse researchers in Canada. The first nurse in Canada to be employed on a full-time basis in a nursing research capacity was Pamela E. Poole, who was appointed as a nursing research consultant by NHRDP in 1965. No current data are available, but in 1977 Storch, Hazlett and Stinson estimated on the basis of their survey of nurses engaged in research in Canada in 1976 that only some six nurses could be classified as full-time nurse researchers at that point in time. This author estimates the 1984 total at approximately 20. (This estimate is exclusive of nurses who are hired as full-time research assistants and/or nurses who collect data for 'medical' and other health related research projects.) The Storch et al. survey identified about 50 nurses who were principal investigators in 1976 (p. 19); this author estimates there were some 450 in 1984. (That estimate includes nurses undertaking a master's thesis or doctoral dissertation.)

In Canada, the term 'nursing research manpower' is applied rather broadly to encompass not only nurses able to design, conduct and report investigations, but also nursing research consultants, and sometimes includes nursing educators and administrators. As yet, Canada has only a handful of nurses who are both expert researchers and expert clinicians, yet there is an increased demand for such people, not only in universities but in the service sector.

PREPARATION FOR RESEARCH

As indicated above, the vast majority (some 85%) of Canadian nurses are 'diploma' graduates from two to three year hospital or community college programs. (The college programs are the predominant type.) Curricula in these programs do not include nursing research courses nor courses in statistics and research design.

While statistics courses have long been a requirement in most undergraduate degree programs in nursing in Canada, courses in nursing research *per se* were introduced only in the '70s. There are

10 master's in nursing programs in Canada, most of which are two years in length, with an emphasis on clinical nursing practice. All such programs require course work in nursing research content and research statistics and design. With one exception, all offer a thesis option and all require a thesis or some type of nursing research project.

The fact that most Canadian master's level nursing programs place great emphasis on research is vitally important as during the next decade, practically speaking, it is those graduates who will continue to occupy the majority of university faculty appointments and/or hold many of the key positions in college and hospital nursing education programs, service agencies, government departments and professional organisations. Thus in Canada, whether they do or do not act as investigators after obtaining their degree, it is important that they have competence in the design and conduct of research, a sound grasp of the major nursing research literature, and advanced literature search skills.

As early as 1976, the Canadian Nurses Association addressed itself to the need for one or more Ph.D. in Nursing programs (Zilm et al., 1979), yet to date, none exists. Thus Canadian nurses undertaking a Ph.D. in Nursing or D.N.Sc. program have done or are doing so in the United States or at the University of Edinburgh (Stinson et al., 1984). The schools of nursing of the University of Montreal and McGill University have proposed a joint Ph.D. in Nursing program, but approval at higher levels, including the provincial government, is as yet to be obtained.[6] The University of Toronto, which has nurses enrolled in their Ph.D. program at the Institute of Medicine, has approved the principle of a Ph.D. in Nursing, but there are as yet no plans for funding this program. More recently, the University of Alberta and University of Calgary Faculties of Nursing jointly developed a proposal to establish a Ph.D. in Nursing program at the University of Alberta by 1986, but it is not yet known if that proposal will be approved and funded by the educational planning authorities.

Given the economic pressures being experienced by Canadian universities and the attendant fact that many Canadian academics do not recognise nursing as a discipline in its own right, education at the doctoral level in nursing promises to be an uphill battle. Yet, in contrast to the mid-'70s, it would seem that it is now not a question of *if* such programs are needed, but only a question of

when and where, and on what bases they will be funded.
Whereas it is not uncommon in the U.K. for nurses to learn to do research primarily by working alongside experienced researchers and undertaking little if any formal research course work, that model is a rarity in Canada. For one thing, there are few career nurse researchers and few extensively funded projects; for another, obtaining university credit for formalised research training is regarded as very important.

For many Canadian nurse researchers, nursing research conferences are the best form of continuing education for research, and for several they are the prime mechanisms for becoming exposed to research. As yet, post-doctoral preparation is a rarity, as are fellowships for full-time post-doctoral research.

ORGANISATION

This author sees two basic dimensions to organisation as it pertains to research: organisation *for research* and organisation *of researchers*.

National Level
While the objectives of the Canadian Association of University Schools of Nursing (CAUSN) and the Canadian Nurses Foundation (CNF) pertain to nursing research, it is the Canadian Nurses Association (CNA) which has been the principal force in organisation *for* nursing research in Canada--even though nursing research development was not made a corporate objective of CNA until 1982. As cited later in this chapter, CAUSN plays important roles in research and education; and the CNF scholarship program has been crucially important in supporting graduate education for nurses. But it is CNA, a federation of all the provincial and territorial professional nursing associations, which has played the prime leadership role over the last decade.

As has been described elsewhere (Stinson, 1977, p. 18), CNA's research role was a rather uneven one up to the early '70s. Then, in 1971, on the heels of the first national nursing research conference, CNA established its first Special Committee on Nursing Research, and maintained such a committee until 1976, when nursing research obtained Standing Committee status. This author regards it as a credit to the vision and commitment

of Canadian nurses, only a few hundred of whom have
direct research experience, to play such a pivotal
role in the development of nursing research.

Another major feature at the national level is
the remarkable extent of cooperation and collaboration amongst CNA, CNF and CAUSN. For example, at
the instigation of CNA, the three organisations
jointly sponsored a national Seminar on Doctoral
Preparation for Canadian Nurses (Zilm et al.,
1979). Based on outcomes of that venture, CNA, in
cooperation with CNF and CAUSN, evolved a five part
nursing research development funding proposal
called 'Operation Bootstrap'. Funding was not
obtained, but the proposal provided an impetus for
research initiatives at the national and provincial
levels.

Collaboration is likely to continue to be an
important characteristic of nursing research development at the national level: the nursing research
community is relatively small; it is not uncommon
for the same nurse to hold office in two or more
national nursing organisations, even at the same
time; the national nursing associations in Canada
tend to be complementary rather than competitive;
and Canadians have a history of considerable interdependence.

Still at the national level, another structural factor of key importance is the National Health
Research and Development Program (NHRDP), not only
in terms of funding nursing research projects but
providing financial support for research training
and for national nursing research conferences. One
of the indirect effects of these conferences is
improved research networking amongst nurses.

The idea of a 'Canadian Council of Nurse
Researchers' was raised at the 1973 national nursing research conference. That idea was further
discussed at the 1975 conference, and hotly debated
at the 1980 conference, held in Halifax. The
controversy still exists and revolves around two
poles: the advantages of a specialised, autonomous
organisation of nurse researchers; and the disadvantages thereof. The prime arguments against
specialised organisation are based on concerns
about divorcing research from nursing as a whole
and that membership would be unlikely to exceed a
few hundred, making it less than viable.

Finally, it should be noted that some of the
clinical nursing specialty organisations at the
national level (e.g. the Canadian Council of Cardio-
vascular Nurses) have established research fellowship and/or scholarship committees and some health-

related national organisations such as the National
Cancer Institute have specific provision for encouraging the development of nursing research.

Regional Level

There are four major political-social 'regions' in
Canada: the Atlantic provinces, Quebec, Ontario and
Western Canada, the latter generally including the
Yukon and Northwest Territories. That is the
structural basis of CAUSN's regional groups. While
the primary focus of CAUSN, both nationally and
regionally, is education, including the development
of an accreditation program for university schools
of nursing, increasing attention is being given to
research, mainly through research papers given at
the national and regional meetings and often
through publication of the proceedings of these
meetings. However, while even ten years ago CAUSN
constituted a logical organisational base for nurse
researchers as most of the nurses conducting research at that time were university faculty members, the same is not true today. Thus, while
CAUSN is significant, its membership is not inclusive enough to constitute a viable base for the
organisation of nursing research or of nurse researchers.

Regional cooperation amongst university
schools in planning graduate education and in
sponsoring national nursing research conferences is
of national significance. However, from the standpoint of nursing research development *per se*,
regional developments are as yet minimal, albeit
that the idea of a Western Consortium for Nursing
Research, instigated by the University of Alberta
Faculty of Nursing, was seriously discussed in the
late '70s. It would appear that regional endeavors
demand that sound *intra*-provincial development
first takes place and/or that interprovincial
collaboration occur within a national rather than
regional context.

Provincial Level

The most striking example of systematic planning
for nursing research at a province-wide level is
that of the Alberta Association of Registered
Nurses, which proposed a beginning 'blueprint'
toward the development of nursing research in
Alberta (AARN, February 1981). In 1981 the Government of Alberta responded by setting aside one
million dollars specifically for nursing research.

To this author's knowledge, and internationally speaking, this is the first time a provincial/state level government has earmarked funds exclusively for nursing research. In October 1982 the Alberta Foundation for Nursing Research was established to administer these funds, over a five-year period.

Another signal development is rooted in the 1980 resolution of the Saskatchewan Registered Nurses Association, that 'it would pay one-half of the cost of a nurse researcher and a secretary for a five-year period to assist in the formation of a Nursing Research Unit at the College of Nursing, University of Saskatchewan.' Initially, recruitment of a Director was a problem, but a nurse researcher was secured for appointment in 1983 (Kyle, personal communication July 15, 1983). The functions of the Unit are somewhat akin to those of the Nursing Research Unit at Edinburgh University, i.e. to serve as a force for nursing research development not only within the University but to have an impact on nursing research in health care agencies as well. Another key intra-provincial development is the emergence of the Manitoba Nursing Research Institute, in 1985, supported by the University of Manitoba and the Manitoba Association of Registered Nurses.

Other examples of development at the provincial level are that in 1982 the Nova Scotia Department of Health approved funding for the staffing of a nursing research unit at the Victoria General Hospital in Halifax, a proposal which involved various nursing groups including the Registered Nurses Association of Nova Scotia and various university faculty members; and by 1982, funding proposals for various types of nursing research units/institutes/consortia had been developed by nurses in cooperation with university schools, the respective provincial professional nursing associations and/or service agencies in British Columbia, Alberta, Ontario, and Quebec.

It would seem fair to say that organisational approaches such as these constitute extraordinary accomplishment and commitment on the parts of the provincial professional nursing associations, the university schools/faculties of nursing, the universities themselves, health care agencies and, in the case of Alberta and Nova Scotia, the provincial governments. And while the above cited examples are 'provincial' in the corporate sense, they are of great national import. Yet Canada has leagues to go in developing a sound infrastructure for nursing research. As has been implied earlier in this chapter, it is often difficult for people from other countries to grasp the vastness of the size of Canada and the sparseness of its population. Outsiders often assume that with its 24 university nursing schools, ten of them with nursing master's programs, the increasing number of nurses with doctoral degrees, etc., Canada should have no trouble moving ahead quickly. But readers should keep in mind the many constraints confronting nursing research development in Canada.

Turning from specific nursing research 'organisations' to province-wide committee structure, another important development over the past decade is the emergence of nursing research committees within the professional provincial nursing associations. There is no direct link between these committees and the CNA's research committee. But they are complementary and interdependent. A survey by the CNA indicates that by 1982 the associations in Alberta, Saskatchewan, Manitoba and Nova Scotia had such committees; B.C. was in the planning stages; Ontario had a member-at-large for nursing research; and that Quebec, P.E.I. and New Brunswick actively supported research in various ways other than through committee structure, a feature true of those with research committees (CNA, June 1982, pp. 2-11). The evidence indicates that much of the work involved reflects immense vision, commitment--and ingenuity.

Thus, by 1982 in the majority of the provinces, some type of *specific* organisation for nursing research had been proposed or was actually operational, whereas 10 years earlier, not a single specific provincial structure existed.

Local Level
The category 'local' is intended here to encompass efforts which may well have national and sometimes even international consequences but which are organised essentially by one or more institutions/agencies within a given location.

Canada has nothing comparable to the well developed, formalised nursing interest groups of the U.K. Prior to the mid 70s, specialised research structure within faculties of nursing was rare, ethics and research committees included. University schools of nursing were the sole organising mechanism for nursing research development. While various types of nursing research interest groups have emerged in the 80s, organisation at the local level is still in its infancy. But there is a qualitative difference from the mid 70s: as more and more nursing research is instigated by nurses employed in health care agencies, nurses 'outside' the universities are gradually becoming integral to what used to be only a university-based nursing research structure. Further, some health care agencies have formed their own nursing research committees, not competitively but in order to give support and visibility to nursing research intra-institutionally. Examples include the Hospital for Sick Children in Toronto and the University of Alberta Hospitals in Edmonton. The definitive trend toward developing positions for nurse researchers within health care agencies' is a generative factor in these respects.

Several initiatives within individual universities or health care agencies are in fact national and even international in their nature and impact. The most striking example is the Centre for Nursing and Health Research, instigated by Dr. Moyra Allen at McGill University and funded through an NHRDP grant. The research conducted by Allen and her colleagues is of international significance.

Within the above context, it will be interesting to see what are the impacts, locally, provincially and nationally, of the newly established Research Facilitation Office of the University of Alberta Faculty of Nursing program, under the direction of Dr. Phyllis Giovannetti, aimed at assisting faculty members and graduate students to develop research funding proposals and disseminate their research findings.

Attention is now directed to international aspects of Canadian nursing research.

International Level
It may at first glance seem a paradox that nursing, organised internationally at such an early date (1899), relative to other professions, lacks specific formalised structure for nursing research. But from a developmental perspective (Stinson, 1969) it is understandable that organisation for service and education would supersede that for research. The questions discussed here are what kinds of organising and organisational roles are Canadian nurses playing in these respects internationally? And how are they affected by nurses and nurse researchers from other countries?

Historically, Canadian nurses have played various roles, directly and indirectly, in the development of nursing research internationally.

Within the United States, the visionary leadership provided by Nutting and Stewart at Teachers College is one such example; Creelman, Girrard, Huffman, Mussallem and Du Mouchel at ICN, Hall of WHO and Cammaert of PAHO are other examples. Then there are those who are 'inherent internationals,' such as Chittick. The points to be made here are that Canadian nurses are not only shaped by international nursing research forces, but to some extent have shaped and are helping to shape nursing research internationally, and in a variety of ways. There being no formalised international structure for nursing research, 'shaping' is largely a matter of communication. The following are specific examples of three types of Canadian involvement:

> *Nursing Research Consultants*: Canada has both utilised and been utilised by nurse researchers from other countries. In the former case are personages such as Simpson, Hockey and Scott-Wright of the U.K.; Wahlberg of Sweden; Henderson, Abdellah, Heidgerken and Lindeman of the U.S.; and in the latter case, nurses such as Allen, Cahoon, Flaherty, Glass, and Giovannetti.

> *National and International Conferences*: Keynote speakers at Canada's first 1971 national nursing research conference included Abdellah and Heidgerken; Simpson from the U.K. was a keynote speaker at the 1973 conference in Toronto, as were Hockey and Hayward from the U.K. and Abbey from the U.S. at the 1975 conference in Edmonton. Literally tens of research presentations have been made by U.S. nurse researchers in Canada at various types of conferences and the same is true for Canadians presenting in the United States. Additionally, Canadians have given nursing research papers in many other countries, including Asia and the Pacific, and at Israel's 1982 International Conference on Nursing Ethics and the Law and three research and research related conferences in Israel in 1985. Canadians have been involved directly and indirectly in a wide range of nursing research endeavors of organisations such as ICN and PAHO (Stinson, 1977, pp. 11-12).
> Some 20 Canadians attended the first international nursing research conference, held in Edinburgh in 1981 (Hockey, 1982), seven of them presenting papers. Three

Canadian nurses gave papers at the 1982 Work-group of European Nurse Researchers (WENR) conference in Uppsala, Sweden (Hamrin, 1983), and eight gave papers at the 1984 WENR-Royal College of Nursing Research Society in London.

Facilitation: Canadian nurses have participated in various conferences and committee work instigated by the International Nursing Interchange of Project Hope, Millwood, Virginia. It was largely through contacts made as a result of those activities that a Canadian was able to construct an inventory of nursing research events of international significance, which facilitated long range planning for such organisations as the WENR, the American Nurses Association (ANA) and the time-tabling of the International Nursing Research Conference to be held in Edmonton, Alberta, May 7-9, 1986. That conference, being sponsored by the Faculties of Nursing of Alberta's three university schools, is being planned in cooperation with the WENR, AARN, and officially endorsed by CNA, CAUSN and the American Nurses' Association, a feature which reflects a sound level of international cooperation. Another example is the internationally important role played by the University of Calgary Faculty of Nursing in sponsoring the International Nursing Informatics Conference, held in Calgary in May, 1985.

Broadly speaking, then, nursing research in Canada is only loosely organised (particularly compared to the U.K.) but the achievements to date are nevertheless of considerable substance, characterised by a cordial tone and by wide scale involvement of all of the major national nursing organisations.

COMMUNICATION

Admittedly, all of the foregoing sections deal implicitly with communication--for nothing would have happened or be happening without it! Again, the author will attempt to provide an overview of the major dimensions of nursing research communication in Canada, using selected examples. Attention is first drawn to the general picture, then to some of the specific aspects of communication.

Basically, the situation in Canada is that mechanisms for communicating nursing research are highly inadequate, as an extract from the CNA Background Paper attests:

Several vehicles for the communication of nursing research activities and findings exist in Canada at the present time. At the local, provincial and national levels, there are organisations and groups that offer the potential for a communication network for nurse researchers and nurses interested in research. At the present time, however, there is little communication between and among these nurses and therefore little co-ordination of effort. Nurses interested in research have expressed a need for some mechanisms to facilitate communication and to disseminate information on research activities and findings.

The Canadian Nurse and *L'infirmiere canadienne*, CNA's two journals, publish news items on research activities, some abstracts of Canadian research studies submitted to the CNA Repository Collection and occasional articles that report research findings. At present, the CNA journals (circulation approximately 129,000) do not have a process of peer-review for articles.... *Nursing Papers*, published by the School of Nursing, McGill University is a peer-reviewed journal that publishes nursing research articles in Canada. However, this journal has a small circulation (approximately 600), and therefore it has a limited audience for the dissemination of research findings. Newsletters published by some provincial nursing associations and special nursing groups also occasionally publish news items on research activities, lists of nursing research titles and abstracts of articles on nursing research studies.

Since 1971, the seven national conferences on nursing research have provided one mechanism for the communication of research through the publication of conference proceedings, and these have contributed to the Canadian literature on nursing research.

The previously-mentioned CNA Repository Collection is a major source of information on completed research; many of the studies in this collection are unpublished master's theses. As this collection depends on the voluntary sub-mission of studies, it cannot be considered a complete collection of Canadian nursing re-search. The Canadian Clearinghouse for Ongoing Research in Nursing [CCORN] at the University of Alberta collects and disseminates informa-tion ongoing projects. It also depends on self-reporting, and requires access to a com-puter for the obtaining of information.

The communication of nursing research through journals, conferences and other vehicles re-mains unco-ordinated and incomplete. There is need for compilation and classification of types and topics of nursing research. (CNA, September 1981, p. 9).[10]

While opportunities within Canada are seriously limited, a mitigating factor is that Canadian nurse researchers do publish (tens of articles yearly) in various nursing and health related research jour-nals of other countries, especially the U.S. and U.K. (e.g. *Nursing Research; Journal of Advanced Nursing; Medical Care; Journal of Health and Human Resources Administration*), as is sometimes the case with textbooks. And to some extent, they publish in journals of other professional and academic disciplines (e.g. *Administrative Science Quarter-ly*).

Impact on Nursing Practice, Education and Adminis-tration
Diers emphasises that the greatest barriers to the actual process of implementing research findings are locating the findings in the first place, and selecting out those which constitute reliable and valid findings (Diers, 1972). There have been no studies in Canada akin to the American Conduct and Utilization of Research in Nursing (CURN) project. We don't *know* how or why Canadian nurses do or do not utilise research. But there is every reason to believe that Canadian nurses have difficulty find-ing research information, as is the situation reported in the CURN project (Loomis, 1982, p. 69). It is the experience of this author that even Canadian nurses prepared at the *doctoral* level are not always highly skilled at locating nursing research literature, particularly if they have studied in other disciplines. There tends to be

heavy reliance on U.S. nursing research literature. The U.S. and to a considerable extent Canadian literature tends to reflect insufficient awareness of related research abroad. And the U.S. literature seldom reflects Canadian nursing research published in English, and almost never reflects that which is published in French.

While the bulk of Canadian nursing research is published in English, much of that published in French is at the vanguard in several respects (e.g. the work of Professor M.F. Thibaudeau and her colleagues at the Université de Montréal). It should be underlined here that both English and French are the official languages of Canada, a feature which on the one hand makes thoroughgoing communication more complex and more expensive but on the other gives richness, breadth, vitality and utility to Canadian nursing research. French is the first language for about one-third of Canadian registered nurses, many of whom are bilingual. Increasingly, unilingual English-speaking nurse researchers are learning to read and speak French.

Networking
While in many ways networking for nursing research in Canada seems considerably effective, there is no literature which even begins to describe the under-lying processes. Prior to the early '70s, there was relatively little research going on, and cross-Canada nursing research networking seemed to depend largely on informal connections between and amongst few people, primarily CAUSN members; the Nursing Consultant for NHRDP; Dr. Helen Mussallem, the then-Executive Director of CNA; CNA presidents, the nursing director of the Canadian Red Cross, Dr. Helen McArthur; and the Principal Nursing Officer (PNO), Verna Huffman Splane. Over the years, PNO's including Huffman Splane, Labelle and now Flaherty have been a potent force in linking various nurse researchers one with another and encouraging nurses to pursue graduate studies. Additionally, by the mid '70s, the CNA research committee constituted a vital networking force, as did the national nursing research conferences -- factors which hold true today.

As the WENR panel at the Uppsala conference attests (Hamrin, 1983, pp. 364-383), one of the most fundamental problems facing nurse researchers, worldwide, is that of communicating, both within and outside the profession. For Canada, it is a pressing problem requiring extensive resources and a high degree of ingenuity.

EPILOGUE

Standing back from this overview it would seem first of all that there is a groundswell for nursing research in Canada -- and a pressing need for an improved infrastructure. Several factors will likely make it difficult for Canadian nursing and nurses to compete for resources for research over the next decade, including the nonscientific image of nurses and nursing. Secondly, it should be emphasised that positive developments in Canadian nursing research are in several respects due to the resources and contributions of people in other countries, and national and international nursing and health-related organisations. Another reality is that for the most part, nursing practice in Canada is still not based on nursing and related research.

As is evident from the literature on professionalisation, professions, like human beings, are shaped by a number of reactive and proactive forces and factors -- and over *time* (Stinson, 1969). In the professional disciplines, research is essentially the third developmental step; service and teaching are normal precursors and ideally all three dimensions develop infinitely. In the case of nursing research, such a perspective leaves no cause for complacency; but neither is there reason for despair. What is amazing to this author about nursing research, both within Canada and worldwide, is not that so much is as yet lacking, but that so much has been achieved under such difficult circumstances -- and in so short a time.

NOTES

1. Virginia Henderson has lamented the fact that the U.S. has produced nothing comparable to the CNA, Royal College of Nursing or the Japanese Nursing Organization libraries. (Personal communication, April 19, 1984.)

2. While it pertains only to Alberta, it is the only inclusive and ongoing inventory of nursing research studies in any province in Canada.

3.   Currently under discussion by MRC.

4.   E.g. the research on infant colic by Dr. Vivian Wahlberg of Sweden in concert with nurse researchers in Italy, the United States and Canada.

5.   Professor J. Gilchrist (Chairman); Dr. H. Glass; Dr. N. Parker; Dr. A. Stark; Dr. S. Stinson; Dr. P. Sullivan; Professor M.F. Thibaudeau. Augmented by a working paper by Professor M. Kyle. The author is indebted to these colleagues for their permission to draw from selected material.

6.   However, one special case Ph.D. in Nursing candidate was approved by McGill University in June 1984.

7.   The first such position was established at the Hospital for Sick Children in Toronto in 1963. (H. Rolstin, personal communication, February 15, 1983)

8.   E.g. of paramount importance to the very fiber of nursing research in Canada is Henderson's monumental *Nursing Studies Index* and the *Survey and Assessment* by Simmons and Henderson (1964), as is the impact of several illustrious U.S. and U.K. nurse researchers and U.S. graduate nursing programs.

9.   Over 560 abstracts from nurses in some 28 countries were submitted for review, an unparalleled number, worldwide. It is expected that this conference will attract 800 to 1000 participants and that it will bring high visibility to nursing research nationally and internationally.

10. Used with permission from CNA.

REFERENCES

Alberta Association of Registered Nurses (1981, February). Toward a blueprint for the development of nursing research in Alberta. Edmonton: Author.

Begin, M. (1983, May). Statement at the Health Ministers' Conference, 36th World Health Assembly, Geneva.

Canadian Nurses Association (1968). *The leaf and the lamp*. Ottawa: Author.

Canadian Nurses Association (1981, September). The development of nursing research in Canada: A background paper. Ottawa: Author.

Canadian Nurses Association (1982, June). Report to Nursing Research Committee. Ottawa: Author.

Diers, D. (1972). Research for nursing. *Journal of Nursing Administration, 2*, 7-12.

Fagin, C. (1982, June). The economic value of nursing research. Paper presented at the Biennial Convention of the American Nurses Association Council of Nurse Researchers. Kansas City, Mo: American Nurses' Association.

Hamrin, E. (Ed.), (1983). *Research - A challenge for practice*. Proceedings of the 5th Workgroup of European Nurse Researchers, Uppsala, Sweden, August 11-14, 1982.

Hockey, L. (1982). *Research - A Base for the Future?* Proceedings of the International Conference, Department of Nursing Studies, University of Edinburgh, September 1981.

Larsen, J., & Stinson, S.M. (1980). *Canadian Nursing Doctoral Statistics*. Ottawa: Canadian Nurses Association.

Loomis, M. (1982). Resources for collaborative research. *Western Journal of Nursing Research, 4*, 65-74.

Medical Research Council. (1985). *Report of the MRC Working Group on Nursing Research*. Ottawa: The Council.

Poole, P.E., & Stinson, S.M. (1974). Some aspects of nursing research in Canada. In D.E. Larsen and E.J. Love (Eds.), *Health care research: A symposium* (pp. 185-188) Calgary: University of Calgary Offset Printing Services.

Simmons, L., & Henderson, V. (1964). *Nursing research: A survey and assessment.* New York: Appleton-Century-Crofts.

Simms, A. (1972). Nursing research in Alberta. Unpublished MHSA project. Edmonton: Division of Health Services Administration, University of Alberta, Edmonton.

Statistics Canada. (1982). *Revised registered nurses data series.* Ottawa: Health Manpower Statistics Section, Health Division, Government of Canada.

Stinson, S.M. (1969). Deprofessionalization in nursing? Unpublished doctoral dissertation. New York, NY: Columbia University.

Stinson, S.M. (1977). Central issues in Canadian nursing research. In B. LaSor & M.R. Elliott (Eds.), *Issues in Canadian nursing* (pp. 3-42) Scarborough, Ontario: Prentice- Hall of Canada Limited.

Stinson, S.M. (1983). How well do managers manage? In Proceedings of *Managing Canada's Health Care System* (pp. 90-102). Financial Post Conference, Saskatoon, Saskatchewan, August 30-31, 1983. Regina: Department of Health.

Stinson, S.M., Larsen, J., & MacPhail, J. (1984). *Canadian nursing doctoral statistics: 1982 update.* Ottawa: Canadian Nurses Association.

Storch, J., Hazlett, C.B., & Stinson, S.M. (1977). *A Canadian survey for nurses engaged in research in 1976.* Edmonton: Division of Health Services Administration, University of Alberta.

Zilm, G.N., Larose, O., & Stinson, S.M. (Eds.), (1979). *Ph.D. (nursing).* Ottawa: Canadian Nurses Association.

Chapter Fifteen

CHRONOLOGICAL ANALYSIS OF NURSING RESEARCH CONTENT
IN AN INTERNATIONAL CONTEXT

Ivo L. Abraham

Every profession expresses concern with its own
future in striving toward the optimisation of
services provided to clients. This concern with
quality improvement is a permanent goal. The means
for achieving this goal can be represented as a
twofold, interdependent process. It is the effort,
on the one hand, to widen theoretical knowledge,
and, on the other hand, to expand usable technolo-
gies. A profession grows by converting its systematically acquired new understanding into new tech-
nologies that will facilitate, if not improve, the
services to be provided.

This philosophical stance is applicable to the
nursing profession as well. The changes within the
profession taking place in various countries over
the world show that nursing is committed to changing its practice as well as improving the grounds
for its practice. Nursing research is emerging as
a reality in many parts of the world, including
Europe.

The purpose of this chapter is to present a
chronological analysis of the European nursing
research movement, and the major issues surrounding
European nursing research development. While major
emphasis is placed on an analysis of trends and
issues as reflected in the literature, this chapter
was written under the assumption that such a chronological analysis is only meaningfully inter-
pretable if its determinants are identified. The
pioneering efforts of international nursing and
health care organisations over the past thirty
years are of paramount importance in this regard.
Selected organisational forces in the advancement
of nursing research are, therefore, first discussed
and the impact of these forces on the methodological focus is described.

The second part of the chapter is an empirical analysis of the scientification of European nursing. A study of the content of 5,035 articles published in eleven nursing journals in four European countries during the years 1976 through 1980 is reported. In this study it was explicitly assumed that trends in nursing publications reflect trends in the profession and that inferences about the past, present, and projections about the future can be made from publication trends. This chapter concludes with a discussion of the process of the scientification of European nursing, as reflected in the empirical analyses outlined in the second part.

Although the chapter is concerned primarily with the European region, and more precisely, with selected West European countries, the author asserts that its applicability and relevance may extend beyond this region. It is not implied, however, that the findings noted for selected countries can necessarily be generalised to all countries in Europe, much less internationally. What is generalisable from this chapter in this author's opinion, is first, the importance of international collaboration across national and cultural boundaries, and the structuring role of formal organisations in such endeavours. Second, using empirical methods of examining publication trends of nursing journals as a means for identifying and defining strands in the advancement (or retrogression) of the profession would also seem of general utility, at least in the Western world. And third, the identified process of scientification of nursing in non-North-American countries without an established research tradition, and the concomitant need to acknowledge cultural, philosophical and scientific traditions when promoting a scientification.

THE ADVANCEMENT OF NURSING RESEARCH IN EUROPE: ORGANIZATIONAL FORCES

A comprehensive description of all the factors that have led to what is now nursing research in Europe is beyond the scope of this chapter. Rather, the content has been limited to a review of major decisions and recommendations regarding nursing and health research as they have been made by international organisations. The endeavours of entities such as the World Health Organization, the International Council of Nurses, and the Workgroup of

European Nurse Researchers have been the major forces in guiding and structuring the work of national nursing organisations in Europe and on building nursing research and theory in these countries.

World Health Organization (WHO)

WHO Expert Committee on Nursing (1966). An Expert Committee on Nursing was formed by WHO in 1966 to study solutions to the increasing quantitative and qualitative demands in nursing services (Farrell, 1983). Among the issues considered by this Expert Group was the encouragement of research in nursing care, services and education.

It was the opinion of the experts that if nursing wanted to meet the challenges of the future, minor modifications of the nursing system would be insufficient. The inevitability of a 'fundamental rethinking' (WHO, 1966, p. 7) was stressed, with a major area of rethinking concerning research as a means of improving nursing practice, nursing services and nursing education. The Expert Group explicitly warned that if research is to serve the profession, 'it must be set within the framework that provides research funds, education that will prepare nurses for research, and means of collating and disseminating research findings' (WHO, 1966, p. 29).

WHO Regional Office for Europe Working Group on Trends in European Nursing Services (1970). The recommendations made by the WHO Expert Committee on Nursing (WHO, 1966) formed the basis for the initiative by the WHO Regional Office for Europe to convene a Working Group on Trends in European Nursing Services (WHO, 1971). This group of nursing administrators, nurse educators, experts in nursing research, and health administrators explored ways of maximising nursing resources for health care. In particular, the participants attended to strategies aimed at adapting nursing practice in European countries to current and future health care needs.

While European countries differ markedly in social organisation and thus in health care systems, one can identify a number of common trends that reflect recent innovations in nursing and in health care delivery. One of them, and probably the most notable one, is the movement directed toward constructing reliable and valid principles for nursing care through nursing research. This indicates that nursing in Europe has come to ac-knowledge that if it wants to exist as a profession and wants to affirm itself as such, it needs to be able to justify its activities. Establishing empirical foundations that sustain the clinical practice is prerequisite to the process of justifi-cation.

It would appear that from the start the Work-ing Group on Trends in European Nursing Services had a major orientation toward empirical approaches in formulating its recommendations as to how nurs-ing services were to be adapted to current and future health care needs. The recommendations were grouped into three categories (1) research and experimentation, (2) education and training, and (3) planning. While the emphasis on research and experimentation might be understandable and even self-evident for American nurses, this was not the case for Europe, as at the time these recommenda-tions were formulated, empiricism as a foundation for clinical practice was a relatively new concept in European nursing.

The following foci of empirical approaches were identified: (i) strategies to raise public awareness and to promote nursing as a career; (ii) the establishment of scientific principles for nursing practice, including standard for quality assurance; and (iii) epidemiological nursing re-search, whereby need models for given population groups are to be constructed.

WHO Regional Office for European Symposia on Nurs-ing Education (1955, 1972). The crucial role assumed by education in the advancement of the nursing profession was acknowledged very early by the WHO Regional Office for Europe. Two initia-tives, a Study Group on Basic Nursing Curriculum in Europe (Note 4) in 1955, and a Symposium on Higher Education Nursing (Note 5) in 1972, are illustra-tive of the Office's stand on these issues.

Even by 1955, the need for research was recog-nised. Indeed, as the proceedings of the 1955 Study Group (WHO, 1955) indicate, there existed among the participants 'a strong feeling ... that recognition of the need for inquiry and investiga-tion in all fields where members of the profession work is a mark of professional status' (p. 40). This early recognition is a possible source of optimism about nursing research in Europe, espe-cially if one considers the following citation from the same proceedings. The Study Group pointed out that 'in addition to the field of treatment, there were unexplored areas of human interactions, human relationships and administrative problems which nurses are in a particularly favourable position to investigate' (p. 40). It was the opinion of participants at both the 1955 (WHO, 1955) and the subsequent 1972 (WHO, 1974) meetings that educational structures be established at the basic and post-basic levels to promote, among other things, nursing research.

WHO Regional Office for Europe Medium Term Programme on Nursing/Midwifery (1976/83). Among the many mechanisms conceived by the WHO to promote health in the world, it organised Medium Term Programmes of limited duration, established periodically, which are of central importance. Each of its five Regional Offices around the world have the autonomy to determine their own programme. Whereas other Regions have elected to attend to issues such as the eradication of selected diseases, the Regional Office for Europe decided to give priority to promoting international collaboration between European countries in nursing and midwifery (WHO, 1977; WHO, 1978).

The European Programme consists of four components: (1) nursing process; (2) organisation and management of nursing services; (3) education and training; and (4) resource planning. Nursing research was considered a key element in implementing the Programme. For this purpose, nine nursing research collaborating centers in eight countries of the Region (Denmark; Finland; France; Netherlands; Poland; Sweden; Switzerland; and Manchester and Edinburgh in the United Kingdom) were set up within existing centers for nursing research. In addition to these, the collaboration of participant centers was obtained, resulting in a vast network of European nursing research centers. Although the impact of this undertaking cannot yet be fully assessed, the evidence indicates that it has to a large extent determined the direction of the expansion of nursing research in Europe.

Other International Organisations
In addition to the considerable efforts of the WHO and its divisions to assist European nursing, two other organisations played important roles. The

contributions by the International Council of Nurses and the Workgroup of European Nurse Researchers are as follows:

<u>International Council of Nurses (ICN)</u>. Although the objectives of the ICN extend world-wide, some of its activities have been particularly influential upon its European member associations and the nurses they represent. The ICN should be considered a forerunner in the advancement of post-basic nursing in the world and in Europe. Between 1951 and 1957, upon request by the WHO and with the assistance of the Florence Nightingale International Foundation (FNIF), the ICN conducted three survey studies on opportunities in post-basic nursing education (FNIF, 1954a; FNIF, 1954b; and FNIF, 1957).

These studies illustrate the concern of the ICN for advanced education for nurses. This interest in nursing research is also apparent from their *Policy Statement on Nursing Research* (reprinted in Lorensen, 1980) which emphasised the facilitation of the conduct of research, but equally its dissemination and utilisation. National nurses' associations were called upon to attend also to the latter two elements of the nursing research process.

It should be added that some thirty years ago, the ICN and the Florence Nightingale International Foundation sponsored two two-week long international seminars in nursing research. The first one took place in Sevres (France) in 1956 (Arnstein & Broe, 1957), the second one was held four years later in Delhi, India (FNIF, 1960). The research endeavours of the ICN continued to grow over the subsequent decades.

<u>Workgroup of European Nurse Researchers</u>. As a result of the WHO Regional Office for Europe Medium Term Programme in Nursing/Midwifery which brought together nurse researchers from all over the Region, the Workgroup of European Nurse Researchers (WENR) has had a pivotal function in the promotion of nursing research in the Region. Being closely associated with the Programme, much of its activities have been linked with those of the Programme. However, this has not restrained members from pursuing their own interests.

The membership of WENR is comprised of one designate from each of the 21 participating national nursing associations. This structure and

limited membership has given rise to some initial
accusations of elitism given that the aim of the
WENR is to promote genuine collaboration in European nursing research. However, it is necessary to
go beyond that criticism of the WENR to appraise
fully the endeavours and achievements of its members. In their respective countries, these members
are in a privileged position to promote the empirical approach. Most of the members are associated
with academic institutions and research centers for
nursing or health care. They maintain close contact with the nursing associations of their countries. Some of them are called upon directly by
their governmental agencies to participate in the
legislative process, or at least function in a
consultative capacity. In short, their expertise
and influence extends over more than one area of
nursing and health care organisation. Their role
in the spreading of the empirical approach in
nursing is commendable.

Summary
A major theme emerging out of this discussion of
organisational forces in the advancement of European nursing is that the WHO, ICN and WENR have
contributed significantly to the pursuit of a
systematic facilitative promotion of a scientific
nursing. The ongoing involvement of these organisations in promoting nursing research reflects,
moreover, recognition of the need for international
collaboration across national, cultural and lin-
guistic boundaries, possibly the major challenge to
European nursing.
The question remains, to what extent the
nursing research related recommendations made
during the past three decades have been implemented, have served their purpose, and have promoted
the profession. This question can best be answered
by examining what nurses and nursing organisations
in Europe have focused on in their professional
endeavours, operationalised in terms of investigating the content of nursing journals in European
countries. If the profession has advanced, one
would expect a solid mass of nursing research and
theoretical papers, a reasonable amount of (preferably empirically supported) clinical articles, and
a relative if not total absence of non-nursing
papers from the cognate disciplines. The next
section of this chapter contains a report on the
analysis of the content of nursing journals in

selected European countries, with major emphasis on research foci.

THE ADVANCEMENT OF NURSING RESEARCH IN EUROPE: AN EMPIRICAL ANALYSIS OF TRENDS AND ISSUES

Purpose of the Study

The study described here originated from a motive to define the current status of nursing in Europe and the directions it took and is likely to take in the future. Since nursing journals assume a pivotal position in the development and growth of the profession, they can simultaneously be regarded as illustrative or reflective of ongoing evolutions. Indeed, one can argue that to the extent that research is not reflected in professional literature, such research is irrelevant in terms of improving nursing practice.

The three major research questions which guided this study were:

(1) What are the publishing trends of European nursing journals in terms of content and clinical nursing domains in focus?

(2) As reflected in nursing journals, what is the current status of nursing in Europe and within European countries?

(3) What importance is attributed to the empirical approach in the development of the profession?

Since a full discussion of the results would exceed the scope of this chapter, attention is first given to overall findings, but the primary emphasis is upon the status of nursing research in selected European countries and trends in nursing research discernible in these countries. It is emphasised here that the findings pertain only to the countries cited, and should not be generalised to all European countries, much less internationally. More particularly, because of this author's inability to comprehend any of the Scandinavian languages, inferences about the status of nursing research in Scandinavia should not be made from this data.

Methods and Procedures

Sample. Because it was impossible to review all journals in all European countries, a selection process was necessary. Selection decisions were based upon two criteria. The first one was the investigator's understanding of the language of publication, and the second one was the completeness of the volumes of the journals available at university libraries in south eastern Michigan (U.S.A.). Moreover, for reasons of manpower and financial constraints, it was necessary to delete one of the two available English journals that are published weekly, *Nursing Mirror* or *Nursing Times*. Since these journals are similar, deletion of one of them was not considered a threat to validity. Random selection indicated that *Nursing Mirror* was to be excluded. Another British journal, *Community Outlook*, was until July 1977 a part of *Nursing Times* but became a small separately published journal. Its data were collapsed with those for *Nursing Times* (NSTIMES). Two international journals, the *International Journal of Nursing Studies* (IJNS) and the *International Nursing Review* (INR), are published in Europe, yet their authorship extends over various countries. Since the focus of the study was to compare selected countries, only those articles whose primary author resided in one of the countries included in the sample were evaluated. This also applied to the British periodical *Journal of Advanced Nursing* (JAN).

Other journals reviewed in this study were: *Midwife, Health Visitor and Community Nurse* (MWHVCN) and *Midwives Chronicle* (MWCHR) for Great Britain; *Revue de l'Infirmiere* (REVUE) and *Infirmiere Francaise* (INF FR) for France; *Deutsche Krankenpflegezeitschrist* (DKPZ) and *Krankenpflege* (KPFL) for West Germany; and *Krankenpflege/Soins Infirmiers* (KP/SI) for Switzerland. Note that until July 1979 the Swiss journal was published under the name *Zeitschrift fuer Krankenpflege/Revue Suisse des Infirmieres*. The major characteristics of these journals are presented in Table 15.1. A total of 5035 articles published during the time period January 1976 - December 1980 was evaluated.

Review Procedures Articles were categorised along three evaluative dimensions: (1) nursing research papers, (2) non-research nursing articles, and (3) cognate contributions without specified relevance to nursing. Moreover, the research articles were classified as either: (a) a research report, (b) a theoretical paper on nursing research, (c) a methodological nursing research article, or (d) a nursing research review. Non-research nursing articles were sub-categorised as: (a) a theoretical nursing article, (b) a clinical nursing article, or

Table 15.1

GENERAL CHARACTERISTICS OF JOURNALS REVIEWED

Country	N*	Journal	n*	Frequency
Great Britain (GB)	3123	NSTIMES	2578	weekly
		MWHVCN	232	monthly
		MWCHR	143	monthly
		JAN	170	bimonthly
West Germany (WG)	938	DKPZ	519	monthly
		KPFL	419	monthly
France (F)	600	REVUE	332	10x/year
		INF FR	268	10x/year
Switzerland (SW)	317	KP/SI	317	monthly
International	57	IJNS	42	quarterly
		INR	15	bimonthly
	5035			

* Number of articles, January 1976 to December 1980.

(c) a nursing education article. Papers from cognate fields were not further differentiated. Because of the nature of this classification system, categorical descriptions needed to be strictly adhered to. These descriptions are summarised in Table 15.2.

Results from a Chronological Perspective

It would be rather meaningless to focus solely on trends in the publication of nursing research articles. The advancement of the profession expresses itself in multiple, interrelated modes. Changes in the conceptualisation of clinical practice, for instance, impose the need for changes in nursing education and have an impact upon professional issues and may generate the need for empirical investigation.

Major Content. Table 15.3 presents an overview of articles published over the five years for each country, and their major content.

No country showed significant fluctuations, be it in an increasing or decreasing direction, for articles with a nursing research orientation. Yet for two countries, West Germany and France, no chi-squared statistic could be computed because of insufficient cell sizes. Note the relatively large proportion of nursing research publications for Great Britain (16.7%) and Switzerland (15.1%) and the minimal such proportion for West Germany (1.6%) and France (1.2%). What these data suggest, then, is that the conduct of nursing research (1) is a function of country/geographical location, and (2) maintained a steady pace (or lack of pace, as in two countries) over the five year period.

Non-research nursing publications showed an increasing trend for West Germany ($X^2(4)=12.82$, $\underline{p}<.02$) and especially for Switzerland ($X^2(4)=20.49$, $\underline{p}<.001$). A status quo was observed for Great Britain and France. Finally, a decrease in cognate publications occurred in Great Britain ($X^2(4)=24.89$, $\underline{p}<.001$) and Switzerland ($X^2(4)=15.83$, $\underline{p}<.001$), yet not in the remaining countries.

A marked conceptual-clinical trend is discernible in these data, as suggested by the decrease in cognate publications in Great Britain and Switzerland, but also by the overall tendency across countries to rely progressively less upon publications from cognate sources ($X^2(4)=29.32$, $\underline{p}<.001$). This effect is largely attributable to trends in

Table 15.2

DEFINITIONS OF MAJOR AND SPECIFIC CONTENT AREAS

Major Content Area	Specific Content Area
NURSING RESEARCH ARTICLE: An article with an empirical orientation and/or purpose that focuses on nursing care and/or health care delivery from a nursing perspective.	(a) Nursing Research Report: research article on one or more clinical and/or educational issues the results of which have implications for clinical nursing practice and/or nursing education and contribute to the enhancement of nursing practice and/or education.
	(b) Theoretical Nursing Research Article: article discussing nursing research as a professional activity and/or discussing certain aspects of nursing research as a component of nursing care and health care delivery; i.e., mainly highlighting the importance, relevance and applicability of nursing research to nursing practice and health care delivery.
	(c) Methodological Nursing Research Article: technical article concerned with methodological and/or statistical issues as they are related to nursing research.
	(d) Nursing Research Review Article: article reviewing the empirical literature on an identified clinical nursing or nursing education topic, or set of topics, with the purpose of summarising and attempting to present a theory, model or concept in clinical nursing or nursing education.

Table 15.2 (continued)

Major Content Area	Specific Content Area
NON-RESEARCH NURSING ARTICLE: An article with a non-empirical orientation and/or purpose that focuses on theoretical, clinical or educational aspects of nursing care and health care delivery from a nursing perspective.	(a) Theoretical Nursing Article: article discussing theoretical aspects of nursing and health care delivery, components of the nursing process, and professional issues. (b) Clinical Nursing Article: an article concerning one or more clinical topics written with the specific intention of enhancing knowledge among and practice of nurses by discussing a concept, method or procedure applicable to nursing practice. The article has to make specific references to nursing implications in order to be considered for this category. (c) Nursing Education Article: an article concerning an educational topic of direct or indirect interest to nursing education written with the specific intent of enhancing nursing education at all levels by discussing a concept, method or procedure that is applicable to nursing education. The relevance to nursing education must be highlighted in order to be considered for this category.
COGNATE ARTICLE: An article concerning a non-nursing topic that does not make specific references to one or more aspects of nursing and	Not further differentiated. Note that specific references to nursing were not present in such articles, i.e., not explicitly formulated.

Chronological Analysis

Table 15.3

MAJOR CONTENT BY YEAR AND COUNTRY

Nursing Research

Country	n	76	77	78	79	80	x^2	df	p<
GB	523	115	95	92	120	101	5.82	4	--
WG	15	3	1	1	4	6			
F	7	5	2	--	--	--			
SW	48	11	7	12	13	5	4.92	4	--

Non-Nursing Research

Country	n	76	77	78	79	80	x^2	df	p<
GB	1593	337	312	319	318	307	1.62	4	--
WG	583	92	111	108	132	140	12.82	4	.02
F	152	28	24	29	31	40	4.69	4	--
SW	214	32	24	44	58	56	20.49	4	.001

Cognate

Country	n	76	77	78	79	80	x^2	df	p<
GB	1052	253	234	215	162	188	24.89	4	.001
WG	341	85	67	75	52	62	9.29	4	--
F	447	89	91	79	96	92	1.80	4	--
SW	60	22	16	5	9	8	15.83	4	.01

Great Britain and Switzerland, yet it should be mentioned that the chi-squared statistic for West Germany ($X^2(4)=9.29$) approached statistical significance at the 0.5 level. Differences were non-significant for France.

Specific Content

Table 15.4 summarises trends over the five year period for each country in terms of the specific content of articles. No country showed significant changes over the years for any nursing research subcategory. Note that Great Britain was the only country with a diversification in nursing research articles, as literature in all four subcategories of nursing research was identified. This is a highly relevant finding. It reflects the level of differentiation attained by Great Britain in its nursing research endeavours. An established nursing research movement is characterised, in this author's opinion, not only by the active conduct of research, but also by the development of specific methodologies for nursing and health research (as indicated by the publication of research methodological papers), and the use of research studies in theory development (hence the publication of research review papers). The publication of theoretical manuscripts on nursing research is considered a final indicator of a differentiated and established nursing research movement. Therefore, the fact that British nurses did publish papers in all four categories is laudable and attests to the status of nursing research in the United Kingdom.

In the category of non-research nursing papers, a trend to emphasise increasingly theoretical nursing papers was observed for France ($X^2(4) = 10.39$, $p< .05$) and Switzerland ($X^2(4) = 15.85$, $p < .01$), whereas West Germany's emphasis appeared to center around publication of clinical papers ($X^2(4)=22.54$, $p<.001$). Articles with an educational emphasis remained at the status quo in all four countries. These findings provide additional evidence for the postulate of a non-cognate conceptual-clinical reorientation in West Germany, France and Switzerland.

Table 15.4

SPECIFIC CONTENT BY YEAR AND BY COUNTRY

Research Report

Country	n	76	77	78	79	80	x^2	df	p<
GB	462	104	85	86	103	84	4.47	4	--
WG	9	2	1	--	2	4			
F	7	5	2	--	--	--			
SW	42	10	7	10	11	4	3.95	4	--

Research Theory

Country	n	76	77	78	79	80	x^2	df	p<
GB	31	5	6	4	7	9	2.39	4	--
WG	6	1	--	1	2	2			
SW	6	1	--	2	2	2			

Research Review

Country	n	76	77	78	79	80	x^2	df	p<
GB	15	2	1	2	4	6			

Research Methodology

Country	n	76	77	78	79	80	x^2	df	p<
GB	15	4	3	--	6	2			

Coun-try	n	76	77	Theory 78	79	80	x^2	df	$p<$
GB	446	81	102	88	92	93	3.13	4	--
WG	123	19	31	22	23	28	3.79	4	--
F	36	3	7	4	8	14	10.39	4	.05
SW	81	10	6	18	25	22	15.85	4	.01

Coun-try	n	76	77	Clinical 78	79	80	x^2	df	$p<$
GB	932	208	108	188	172	184	3.88	4	--
WG	333	49	49	61	84	90	22.54	4	.001
F	105	23	16	23	21	22	1.62	4	--
SW	108	18	15	20	26	29	6.17	4	--

Coun-try	n	76	77	Educational 78	79	80	x^2	df	$p<$
GB	215	48	30	43	54	40	7.53	4	--
WG	127	24	31	25	25	22	1.78	4	--
F	11	2	1	2	2	4		4	
SW	25	4	3	6	7	5	2.00	4	--

Summary
Findings across countries are difficult to summarise because of the substantial differences between Great Britain and the other three countries. Publishing trends in Great Britain appeared to have attained an established pattern which, because of the large output, had a stabilising effect on the less consistent data of other countries.

A decrease was found in the article output per year for Great Britain, but the rate for West Germany, France and Switzerland was consistent. The major content of the publications pointed at a conceptual-clinical redirection for the three continental countries, yet such a level had already been attained by Great Britain. Findings pertaining to manuscripts from a cognate source supported this contention, as did the data for specific content. Great Britain appeared to be ahead in nursing research even in 1976, and this did not significantly alter over the years in any specific content area. This finding was in contrast with the other countries where, with the exception of Switzerland, a lack of nursing research was observed. Finally, the trend to address issues in clinical nursing and divert from cognate publications irrelevant to nursing practice was definitive.

The question remaining is the extent to which these trends of the past are likely to extend into the future.

Prediction of Trends Through Log-Linear Models
For a long time there were no adequate statistical procedures for constructing models or equations from nominal data. Model construction and prediction were reserved for internal and ratio data by application of regression analysis.

Log-linear analysis, a statistical procedure recently being applied in the social sciences, has received increasing attention especially from political scientists (Reynolds, 1977). In contrast with regression analysis, log-linear analysis does not utilise individual scores but mathematical functions of cell probabilities. The most widely used mathematical function is the natural logarithm ($\ln$) which has the natural number ($e=2.7182818$) as basis. Log-linear analyses have allowed social scientists to measure and test uni- and multivariate tabulations of cell frequencies.

This study entailed assessing existing trends and determining the likelihood that they would

manifest themselves in the future. Log-linear
analyses were performed to assess the goodness of
fit of equations that aimed at modelling the frequency of publication of articles in general, of
nursing research papers, non-research nursing
papers, and cognate manuscripts. Equations were
developed and tested along these dimensions for
each individual country.

The goodness of fit of a model is indicated by
the coefficient of determination R^2, which is the
correlation coefficient to the second power. Since
the distribution of R^2 follows an exponential
function, units of increase or decrease are not
necessarily equal. Although in many instances an
R^2 of .35 is considered sufficiently large, in this
study .45 was used as standard. Because of the
relatively short period of time covered by this
study, it was decided to approach predictions
conservatively. R^2 can be interpreted best as the
percentage of variation in the data that is accounted for by the model.

A log-linear analysis for a tabulation of
nominal data uses the natural logarithm ln of the
cell frequencies and constructs equations in which
the predicted value, slope and intercept are expressed as natural logarithms. Utilising the
natural logarithm instead of the actually observed
frequencies compensates for the assumption of
normality in distribution which is nonexistent for
nominal data. Moreover, it accounts for the fact
that data such as those reported here might satu-
rate at some point. It is indeed difficult to
imagine that, if a model suggests that an increase
in, for example, research articles is likely, this
increase will manifest itself into eternity. Thus,
the natural logarithm takes into account that data
follow an asymptotic curve of saturation.

The log-linear model utilised in this study
was of the following general form:

$$\ln Y = \ln a + \ln b(X)$$

with lnY being the predicted natural logarithm of
the frequency; lna the natural logarithm of the
intercept; lnb the natural logarithm of the slope;
and X the year of publication.

Log-Linear Analyses for Article Output
Figure 15.1 portrays the models for predicted
overall output. Accurate models were constructed
for Great Britain, West Germany and Switzerland.

The model for Great Britain ($\underline{\text{ln}}a$ = 9.57; $\underline{\text{ln}}b$ = .04), explained 87 percent of the observed variation. Similarly, 82 percent of the variation for West Germany was accounted for by its log-linear model ($\underline{\text{ln}}a$ = 2.54; $\underline{\text{ln}}b$ = .03). The Swiss model yielded a $\underline{R}^2$ = .45 ($\underline{\text{ln}}a$ = -3.08; $\underline{\text{ln}}b$ = .09). No sufficiently accurate model could be constructed for France.

Figure 15.1 suggests that by 1990, a convergence in overall output of articles in the different countries can be expected. This entails a predicted decline in output for Great Britain, and a predicted incline for West Germany and Switzerland.

Log-Linear Analyses for Nursing Research Papers

Because of insufficient cell frequencies, no analyses were performed for West Germany and France. It will be recalled that in these countries nursing research articles accounted for respectively 1.6 and 1.2 percent of total article output. Furthermore, neither for Great Britain nor for Switzerland could accurate models be constructed. The British model yielded a $\underline{R}^2$ = .024. The Swiss model yielded a $\underline{R}^2$ = .14.

The finding that no prediction for nursing research in Europe can be made could conceivably be interpreted as an undesirable and discouraging finding from a professional advancement perspective. However, it must be underlined that the insufficient cell frequency problem does not permit any definitive interpretation in these respects.

Log-Linear Analyses for Non-Research Nursing Papers

In contrast with research papers, highly accurate models were developed for non-research nursing papers (see Figure 15.2). The most accurate model, accounting for 91 percent of the variance, was constructed for West Germany ($\underline{\text{ln}}a$ = -3.13; $\underline{\text{ln}}b$ = .1), followed by Switzerland ($\underline{R}^2$ = .70; $\underline{\text{ln}}a$ = -11.74; $\underline{\text{ln}}b$ = .2) and France ($\underline{R}^2$ = .68; $\underline{\text{ln}}a$ = -4.1; $\underline{\text{ln}}b$ = .1). The British model explained 52 percent of the observed variance ($\underline{\text{ln}}a$ = .01; $\underline{\text{ln}}b$ = .02).

These models revealed that non-research nursing documents are increasingly receiving priority, thus suggesting a trend to expand the theoretical-clinical knowledge base of nursing. Although the British model predicted a decline in this category of articles, this can be ascribed to either

Figure 15.1

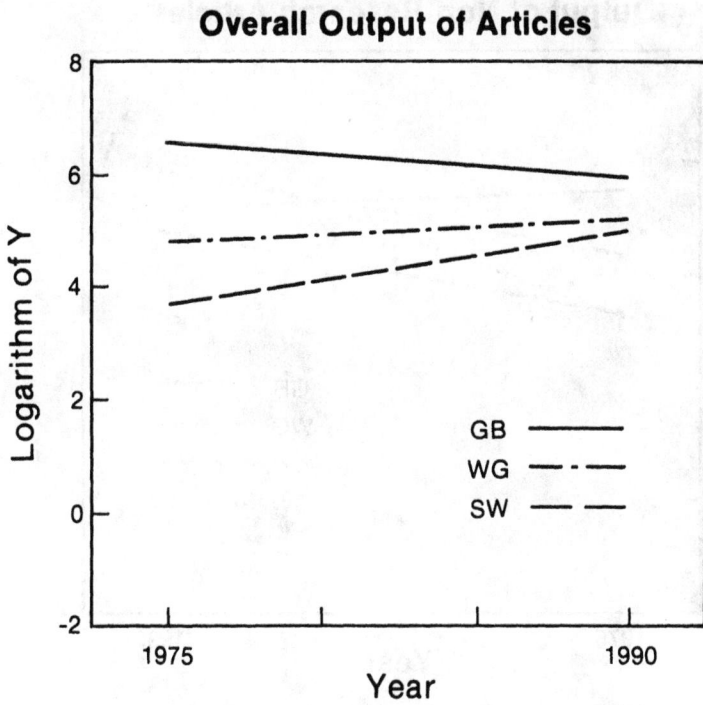

Overall Output of Articles

Figure 15.2

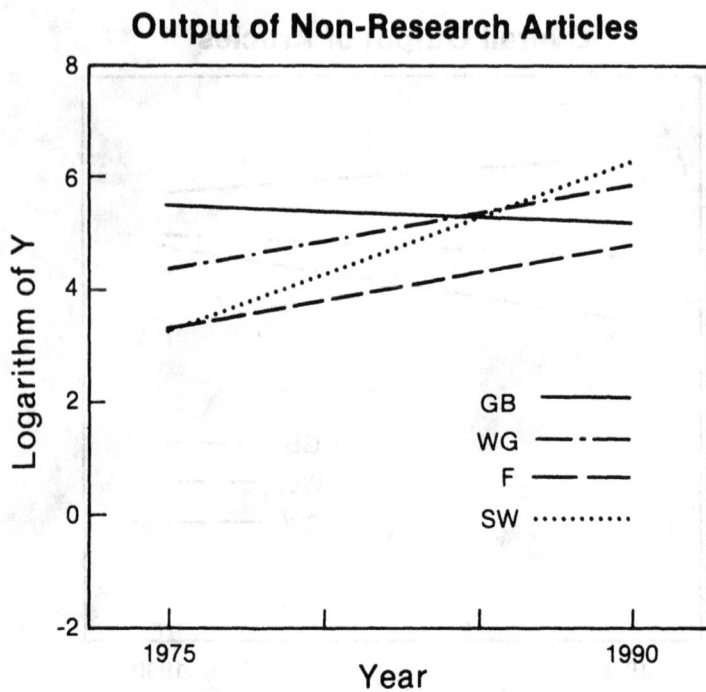

Output of Non-Research Articles

the general decrease in this type of output observed for this country, or to mere chance.
 The trend noted for Switzerland, France and
West Germany will not necessarily culminate in a
convergence as was observed for overall output.
The West German and French models have equally
increasing slopes, which are however less pro-
nounced than the slope, and thus unit of increment,
in the Swiss model. It is thus justifiable to
assume that West Germany, France and Switzerland
will further develop a clinical-conceptual direction, yet at a different pace.

Log-Linear Analyses for Cognate Papers
It was mentioned earlier in this chapter that, in
general, journals were found to rely decreasingly
upon publications from cognate sources. Figure
15.3 suggests that this trend will continue in all
countries except France. Great Britain's model
yielded a R^2 = .72 (lna = 12.67; lnb = -.09). A
similar slope (lnb = -.9) was found for West Germany (lna = 10.99; R^2 = .54). The strongest decline
is expected to occur in Switzerland where the slope
equalled -.26 (lna = 22.55; R^2 = .49).
 These findings lend additional support to the
contention that European nursing journals are
likely to pursue a conceptual-clinical, nonempiri-
cal, direction. Attention is now directed to an
elaboration of that contention.

TOWARDS A SCIENTIFICATION OF EUROPEAN NURSING

The Past as Basis for the Future
Where is nursing research likely to stand in relation to these factors in the future? The data may
reflect a grim situation, with the exception of
Switzerland and Great Britain. The Scandinavian
countries, although not a part of this study, may
be counted under this exception as well (Hamrin,
1983). Yet, in general, the conclusion that nursing research is and for some time may remain the
forgotten contributor to the advancement of nursing
in Europe seems warranted, especially in the Roman-
ic (France, Italy, Spain, Portugal, and Francophone
Belgium) and the Germanic countries (West Germany,
Austria, and to an extent, Dutch-speaking Belgium
and the Netherlands).
 It would be a mistake to infer from this
relative lack of research activity that nursing in

Figure 15.3

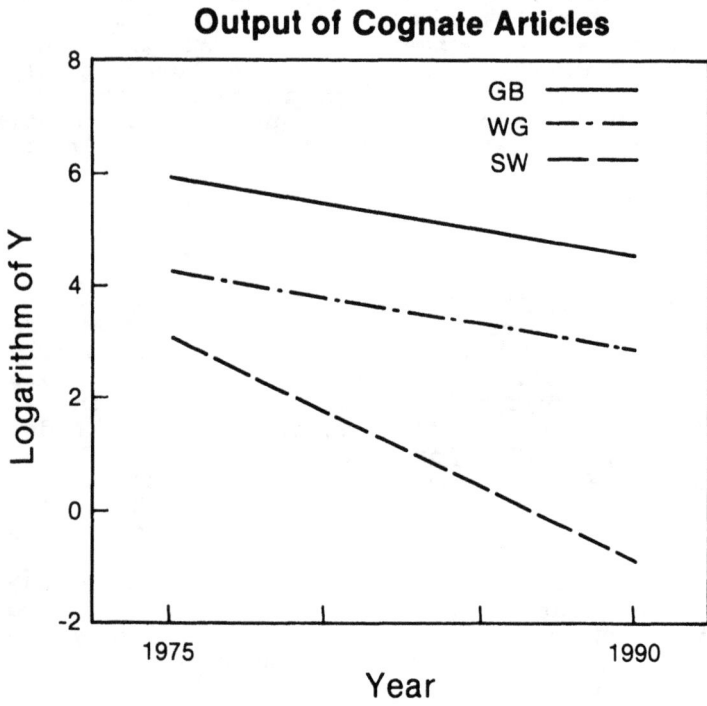

Output of Cognate Articles

Europe is behind and, moreover, not in a position to move ahead, for in many of these countries there are strong indicators that the profession *is* advancing. There is, for instance, the network of research centers developing during the WHO Medium Term Programme for Nursing/Midwifery. Many countries now offer opportunities for advanced nursing education, with most of them featuring a research component. France, with its advanced nursing program affiliated with the Universite de Lyon has moreover contributed to the advanced education of non-French nurses from several countries in Europe and the Third World. Also, in the summer of 1982 the first Open Conference of the Workgroup of European Nurse Researchers was held in Uppsala (Sweden); and planning for biennial WENR conference is well under way. The 1984 Conference was held in London in April 1984 in concert with the Royal College of Nursing. Many other examples to support the theme that the profession is advancing, albeit slowly in research, can be cited.

It is emphasised that, in this author's opinion, the current situation is *not at all negative*. On the contrary, not only is nursing research investigation being promoted and facilitated, but attention is being given to the dissemination and utilisation of nursing research findings. In this way, some of the mistakes which seem to have been made in the development of the American nursing research movement can be prevented. We refer hereby to the over-enthusiasm which seemed to engulf American nursing scholars in the sixties and early seventies, which resulted in a massive production of research without sufficient attention to its integration into clinical practice. European nursing is less likely to create a research movement divorced from clinical practice (Prophit, 1982).

Even if the data reflect some findings which could be given a negative interpretation, they suggest a *positive theme* in European nursing. Even over the short five year period covered by this study, one can observe an evolution in the conceptualisation of nursing. The trend towards recognising nursing as a clinical discipline with a theoretical foundation is a definitive one. This foundation, or knowledge base, is as of yet theoretical-hypothetical: assumptions about nursing must be validated by personal conviction and *a priori* theorisation, rather than simply by more objective research approaches. From a European and thus non-American perspective, such an orientation is very understandable. European thinking has been strongly structured by Cartesian thinking, whereby preference is given to *a priori* theorisation and a subsequent deductive empirical validation. This cultural property must be taken into account when promoting nursing and nursing research in Europe.

In summary, there is sufficient evidence to support the proposition that nursing in Europe is reconsidering and reshaping its professional content. A commitment to scientification appears to be well established.

The Scientification of European Nursing: The Theoretical-Hypothetical versus Theoretical-Empirical Knowledge Base

The necessity of creating an empirical foundation for clinical practice is receiving increasing recognition. However, this foundation is as of yet primarily theoretical-hypothetical in nature as opposed to being of a theoretical-empirical type.

It would be a mistake to assume that European nursing is, therefore, missing the boat of empiricism. First, specific cultural and social characteristics need to be fully appreciated, as emphasised above. Secondly, the unavailability of, or at least paucity of, nursing research funding to date is another factor. Thirdly, the observed theoretical-hypothetical approach is not a direction which is opposite to the theoretical-empirical one; on the contrary, it is an evolutionary component in the process of scientification.

Indeed, the theoretical-hypothetical orientation is essential in nurses becoming acquainted with scientific models of thinking. Simultaneously, it permits the profession to begin identifying problems and issues which are in need of empirical validation. It is this author's contention, then, that the scientification of European nursing is in its 'next-to-last' phase. Figure 15.4 visually presents a model of the scientification process of European nursing.

It is acknowledged that this model is in contrast with the actual evolution of the nursing profession in the United States, where the empirical approach preceded the theoretical-hypothetical stage. The need for nursing research was already being emphasised when in fact there was a lack of *identified* researchable questions. This is understandable from a cultural perspective in that inductive thinking (as opposed to deductive, Cartesian thinking) is much more predominant in the

Figure 15.4

The Scientification Process

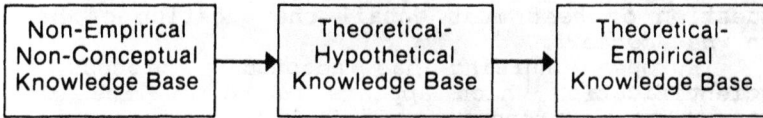

| Non-Empirical Non-Conceptual Knowledge Base | → | Theoretical- Hypothetical Knowledge Base | → | Theoretical- Empirical Knowledge Base |

United States. It is also understandable if one considers that in the American scientific and academic community research assumes a position of high priority, and that professional advancement in the academic community is primarily a function of scholarly productivity.

It is simplistic to imply that one can or should evaluate which approach is *best* since the question of *best* must entail the question of best *in what context.*

European nursing has adopted a process of scientification which appears to be in line with its cultural properties, and from a sociological perspective, that would seem *best* within that cultural context.

A final issue concerns how European nursing can successfully further develop a culturally congruent research movement. It is contended here that if European countries want to develop further nursing research they will not only need to create a movement of *doing* research, but equally a movement of *collecting, adopting,* and, if necessary, *adapting* previously conducted studies. Those countries without an established nursing research tradition should utilise previous theoretical-hypothetical and theoretical-empirical research and build upon it. There are in nursing so many areas untouched by research yet in need of attention. This then calls for a collaboration between countries without a nursing research tradition, and countries with such tradition. Such concerted effort will aid in the attainment of the ultimate objective: the establishment of a truly international nursing research movement.

In conclusion, the present of European nursing research may not be what the nursing profession wishes it to be; yet it is clearly in a state of expansion. Further, this author believes that European nursing research and its efforts to co-ordinate multiple countries, with varied languages and cultural kaleidoscopes, will ultimately be as successful as nursing research in the United States, with its one language and country.

NOTES

The author wishes to thank Judy Ozbolt and Susan Boehm for their comments on earlier versions of this chapter. The writing of this chapter also benefited from the conversations during the past two years with (in alphabetical order) Lois Gage,

Elizabeth Hamrin, Sr. Penny Prophit, and correspondence with Marie Farrell. The responsibility for the content of this chapter, however, rests solely with the author.

REFERENCES

Arnstein, M.G., & Broe, E. *(1957)*. *International conference on planning of nursing studies*. London: International Council of Nurses/Florence Nightingale International Foundation.

Farrell, M. (1983). Personal communication. Letter received March.

Florence Nightingale International Foundation. (1954). *An international list of advanced programmes in nursing education (1951-1952)*. London: International Council of Nurses.

Florence Nightingale International Foundation. (1954). *How to survey a school of nursing: A suggested method, illustrated with samples of five post-basic schools*. London: International Council of Nurses.

Florence Nightingale International Foundation. (1957). *Post basic nursing education: Principles of administration as applied to advanced programmes in nursing education*. London: International Council of Nurses.

Florence Nightingale International Foundation. (1960). *Learning to investigate nursing problems*. London: International Council of Nurses.

Hamrin, E. Personal communication. (1983). Ann Arbor, U.S.A., June.

Lorensen, M. (Ed.), (1980). *Collaborative research and its implementation in nursing*. Copenhagen: Danish Nurses Association.

Prophit, P., Sr. (1982). Personal communication. Leuven, Belgium, July.

Chronological Analysis

Reynolds, H.T. *(1977)*. *Analysis of nominal data.* Sage University Paper Series on Quantitative Applications in the Social Sciences, series no. 07-001. Beverly Hills & London: Sage Publications.

World Health Organization Regional Office for Europe. (1955). *Study group on basic nursing education.* Geneva: WHO Regional Office for Europe.

World Health Organization Regional Office for Europe. (1971). *Trends in European Nursing Services: Report on a Working Group.* Copenhagen: WHO Regional Office for Europe.

World Health Organization Regional Office for Europe. (1974). Symposium on higher education in nursing: Summary report. *Archives Belges de Medicine Sociale, Hygiene, Medicine de Travail et Medicine Legale/Belgisch Archief van Sociale Geneeskunde, Hygiene, Arbeidsgeneeskunde en Gerechtelijke Geneeskunde*, 32, 167-172.

World Health Organization Regional Office for Europe. *(1978)*. *Medium Term/Programme on Nursing/Midwifery in Europe (1976-1983).* Copenhagen: WHO Regional Office for Europe EURO/NURS/78.2.

World Health Organization Regional Office for Europe. (1978). *Medium Term/Programme on Nursing/Midwifery in Europe: Implementation of phase 2.* Copenhagen: WHO Regional Office for Europe EURO/NURS/78.2.

World Health Organization, WHO Expert Committee on Nursing, fifth report. (1966). *World Health Organization Technical Report Series*, no. 347.

Chapter Sixteen

THE AMERICAN NURSES' ASSOCIATION: ITS ROLE IN
NURSING RESEARCH

Pauline Brimmer

Since its establishment in 1896, the American
Nurses' Association (ANA) has gathered data on
nurses. Recognising the importance of these data
to the profession, the House of Delegates, as early
as 1946, approved certain well-defined objectives
including the expansion of the research and statistical capabilities of the association. One of the
activities under this objective was the completion
of studies of nursing functions which was approved
as a five-year program of research by the House of
Delegates in 1950. It became clear as this program
evolved, that there were other needed areas of
research consistent with the aims and purposes of
the ANA and in the public interest. Since these
needed studies would be costly, the ANA Board of
Directors did not feel that membership dues could
be used for this purpose. Subsequently, the American Nurses' Foundation (ANF) was established and
other sources of funds, that could be tax free
contributions, were solicited for research. Another emphasis for research in the association occurred at the 1958 convention from goals established by the Current and Long-Term Goals Committee
of the American Nurses' Association.
The committee's supplemental report stated:

A major focus of the committee's discussions
has been on the broadened concept of nursing as
an intellectual discipline with a specific body
of knowledge. It recognises that the scientific bases of nursing knowledge may be derived
from many of the physical and social sciences
and, insofar as these sciences have unique
applications in nursing, they become the basic
intellectual identity of the profession. The

ANA Committee on Current and Long-Term Goals
has concluded that improvements and changes in
the practice of nursing should primarily result
from enlargement and refinement of this body of
knowledge. With this as a basic premise, the
committee believes that the future of nursing
should increasingly be dependent upon the
results of research in nursing undertaken by
nurses themselves (ANA Convention Proceedings,
1958, p. 70).

Also discussed by this committee was the lack
of nurses educated in research, and the need for
special educational preparation for nursing students who choose research careers. Two goals were
presented by the committee for long-range planning.
The first goal was for the stimulation of nursing
research and its application in practice. The
Cabinet[1] on Nursing Research initiated in 1970 and
the Council of Nurse Researchers established in
1971 have worked diligently to implement this goal.
The second goal was to establish ways within ANA to
provide formal recognition of personal achievement
and superior performance in nursing. From this
second goal, the impetus developed to establish the
American Academy of Nursing (AAN) in 1973 which
challenges current practices and encourages innovative ideas for change.

These three bodies, ANA, ANF, and AAN, opened
the door for the advancement of the nursing profession and the development and the dissemination of
nursing knowledge. By their initiative and future
orientation, they became a driving force for nursing research in the United States.

ANA, ANF, and AAN are closely related, and
this interrelationship will be apparent in this
chapter. The first part of the chapter is a discussion of the ANA and research activities since
1978; the second and third parts discuss ANF and
AAN respectively. The conclusion briefly reports
on the collaboration between ANA and the other
organisations, and between ANA and state research
groups. The discussion of the establishment of a
Center for Research at ANA sets future directions
for research and research activities within the
association.

AMERICAN NURSES' ASSOCIATION (ANA)

ANA has had a long and evolving history, since the
early 1950s, in conducting and supporting research
and research activities. For a chronology of
events which highlight the development of these
activities and the increasing priority research and
research support have received from ANA since that
time until 1978, read See, 1977, and Brimmer, 1978.
Only the work of ANA in the research arena from
1978 will be discussed here.

Department of Research and Policy Analysis
For more efficient functioning of headquarters
staff, consolidation of certain units and departments became necessary in 1979. In July, the staff
of the Department of Research, Grants, and Contracts; the Human Rights Unit; and the position of
manpower economist were merged to form the Department of Research and Policy Analysis. In September, the Department of Statistics also became part
of this new department. The purpose of the Department of Research and Policy Analysis is to implement a co-ordinated strategy for development of
association policies relative to nursing personnel,
the nursing profession, and the human rights of
nurses and consumers by using statistics, manpower
analysis, and research. Department staff also
provide support services for ANA's Cabinet on
Nursing Research and Council of Nurse Researchers
and their related committees. In addition, staff
provide support for ANA's Institutional Review
Board; Cabinet on Human Rights; and function as
project officer for the American Nurses' Foundation. During the 1980-1982 biennium, ANA moved to
expand its data base on the economics and practice
characteristics of nurses. The ANA Office of Labor
Research was established in Washington, D.C., and
an economic policy analyst was appointed to the
Kansas City research staff.
   Two major statistical projects undertaken by
staff in 1978 and 1979 were the 1977 national
sample survey of registered nurses (Roth, Graham &
Schmittling, 1979) and the 1977-1978 registered
nurse inventory (Schulte, 1981). Both of these
projects were federally funded. Staff compiled and
the American Journal of Nursing Company published
the 1980-1981 *Facts About Nursing* (ANA, 1981a). A
study of nurses with doctoral degrees, funded by
the Division of Nursing, Public Health Service,
began September 1, 1978. As part of the study, a

directory of nurses with doctoral degrees was published by ANA in 1980 (ANA, 1980). The total project was completed in 1981, and articles are in process for publication or are being prepared for publication in major nursing journals.

The first issues of a monograph series concerned with economic and employment issues of nurses were published in November, 1982. Ten issues per year are planned. Staff are also monitoring the supply and demand for nurses, and began a monthly index of the demand for nursing services in 1983.

Cabinet on Nursing Research

Accomplishments of the Cabinet on Nursing Research since 1978 were consistent with its goals. The commission completed a five-year plan for the expansion of the ANA intramural research program. As part of that plan, a policy for the review of proposed intramural research was developed and guidelines were provided for access to ANA data files for secondary analysis.

Since the cabinet was instrumental in developing and guiding the study of nurses with doctoral preparation, it maintained continual communication with the steering committee of the project, 'Nurse Doctorates: A National Information System Model'. Plans were made to update the directory of nurses with doctorates every three years and the total data file every six years.

The Cabinet on Nursing Research developed and maintained relationships with federal officials and presented testimony before various federal groups. A major goal was to strengthen support of nursing research at the federal level. Two subcommittees of the cabinet co-ordinated initiatives in that arena. The Legislative Coordinating Committee worked with members and staff of the U.S. Congress, and the Administrative Liaison Subcommittee directed its attention to federal administrative agencies. During the 1978-1980 biennium, the Legislative Coordinating Committee developed a national network, called the Legislative Action Subcommittee, to maintain ongoing relationships with legislators at the state level. Most of the 50 states and the District of Columbia have one representative for research who has set up a local/state network of nurses for influencing legislators.

During the 1980-1982 biennium, in cooperation with the Extramural Research Office, National Institutes of Health (NIH), and with other agencies

of the United States Public Health Service (PHS),
the cabinet offered an opportunity for nurse researchers to participate in an unusual program.
The program was designed to help nurse investigators who lacked a research track record have draft
proposals reviewed and get to know at least one
staff member in a relevant NIH or other PHS agency.
One hundred and ten proposals from 28 states were
received and distributed to 11 agencies of the
federal government. Staff personnel in the various
research funding agencies reviewed and critiqued
the proposals. Critiques were sent to the individual researchers. Opportunities were then provided
by the cabinet for these individual researchers to
visit agency personnel while at the 1982 convention
in Washington, D.C. With the constructive criticism and personal visits, full-fledged proposals
with funding potential could be prepared by the
nurse investigators and submitted for possible
approval.

The cabinet reviewed the need for a taxonomy,
investigated the status of international nursing
research, and began to develop plans for increasing
private support for nursing research. The cabinet
participated in planning the 1979 clinical and
scientific sessions held in Nashville, Tennessee in
November, and co-sponsored program presentations
with the ANA Division on Gerontological Nursing
Practice. Cabinet programs were also presented at
the Council of Nurse Researchers' annual conference
and at the ANA conventions.

As requested by the ANA Board of Directors, in
relation to the 1982-1984 biennium, the Cabinet on
Nursing Research selected the association priority
that it could most effectively address during that
biennium: expand the knowledge base for the practice of nursing through research, the major strategy being to continue stimulating research activities in practice, service, and educational settings. To implement this strategy, the cabinet
addressed itself to a policy statement that sets
forth a plan for nursing research in the twen-
ty-first century. The statement is intended to
provide direction for the conduct of research and
preparation of researchers in the coming decades.

Another approach to implementing the selected
strategy is developing policies to promote information exchange and collaboration between ANA and
state nurses' associations (SNA's) with research
structures. As ANA implements the modified federation model, this becomes critical. To promote
exploration of ANA-SNA working relationships in the

area of research, the cabinet then planned a program focused on state research.

Publications of the Cabinet on Nursing Research include: (a) *Nursing Research: Synopsis of
Selected Clinical Studies* (ANA, 1979) developed to
delineate the types of research undertaken by
nurses seeking to develop a scientific basis for
practice; (b) *Research Priorities for the 1980s:
Generating a Scientific Basis for Nursing Practice*
(ANA, 1981b) which gives a definition of nursing
research and directions for nursing research; and
(c) *Guidelines for the Investigative Functions of
Nurses* (ANA, 1981c) which delineates the research
activities appropriate to nurses prepared in different types of educational programs. Work has
been completed for a fourth publication, 'Selecting
a Doctoral Program with an Emphasis on Research
Preparations'. Plans are in process to update
*Research in Nursing: Toward a Science of Health
Care* (ANA, 1976) and *Human Rights Guidelines for
Nurses in Clinical and Other Research* (ANA, 1975).

Liaisons are maintained by the Cabinet on
Nursing Research with various structural units of
ANA, the American Academy of Nursing, the American
Nurses' Foundation, the American Association of
Colleges of Nursing, and others in order to deter-
mine opportunities for collaborative effort.
Liaisons also continue with the National Institute
of Medicine and various federal agencies to inter-
pret the need for nursing research and to seek
resources.

Council of Nurse Researchers

The Council of Nurse Researchers continues to
address the scientific priorities of the profession
and the research needs of the constituency. Two
statements were prepared by the executive committee
of the council at the request of the American
Nurses' Foundation. The first was the development
of a rationale for providing research assistance to
developing countries. The second was drafting
criteria for the Distinguished Contribution to
Nursing Science Award and developing the procedure
for selecting the individual to be honored by the
American Nurses' Foundation. This award has been a
long standing goal of the Council of Nurse Researchers.

A call for nursing abstracts was issued
through the quarterly newsletter of the Council of
Nurse Researchers. These were to be compiled and
published to inform nurse researchers of current

investigations. Because of budgetary limitations, abstracts were not published, but they have been used as a source for selecting expert witnesses for testimony before state and federal organisations.

The executive committee of the council collaborated with the ANA Cabinet on Nursing Practice to plan and present a conference in 1979 on evaluation research. This invitational conference was planned as a bridge between practice and research, with a priority being the use of research findings in practice. Major papers presented at the conference were published in the March-April 1980 issue of *Nursing Research*. A follow-up program on evaluation research was presented at the 1980 ANA convention.

Criteria have been developed to be used in considering the names of individuals to serve as members of peer review and public advisory committees. The executive committee periodically reviews names with the criteria so that nurses will be available for consideration as vacancies occur.

Over 275 participants attended an October 1982 conference in California sponsored by the ANA Council on Continuing Education, Council on Nursing Administration, Council on Intercultural Nursing, and the Council of Nurse Researchers. This conference on networking offered many opportunities for strengthening existing networks and establishing new ones for the advancement of nursing.

Annual conferences and business meetings were held each year, at the ANA conventions in 1980, 1982 and 1984, and independently in 1979 and 1981. A conference was held in Minneapolis, Minnesota in September 1983, with the theme, 'Nursing Science: Today and Beyond.' The purpose of the conference was summarized as identifying the current state of the science and future directions for nursing research. The conferences usually host approximately 400 people and include awards to new and established investigators. The ANA Council of Nurse Researchers is also presently involved in planning for an international nursing research conference to be held in 1987. The focus of this conference will be nursing's advances in health.

By emphasising recruitment the council doubled its membership by the early 80's to some 700 members. Further, the quarterly *Council of Nurse Researchers Newsletter* is widely circulated and is growing in volume and popularity.

Liaisons are maintained with structural units of ANA and various external organisations with research as their focus. Representatives of the council attend state and federal meetings and give testimony as needed.

The last few years have been productive ones in the area of research for the Department of Research and Policy Analysis, the Cabinet on Nursing Research, and the Council of Nurse Researchers.

AMERICAN NURSES' FOUNDATION (ANF)

ANF is a vigorous and flourishing foundation, separately incorporated, but working closely with ANA. The foundation focuses its efforts in three basic areas: (a) support for the career development of nurses by funding research projects; (b) the analysis of health policy issues of major concern to nursing; and (c) assistance to the educational and research activities of ANA. In pursuing these three activities, ANF is carrying out the major functions for which it was established by ANA some 30 years ago.

Establishment of a Foundation

The 1954 ANA biennial convention proceedings include a statement that a major philanthropic organisation had offered ANA significant funds for a project consistent with the aims and purposes of ANA. Unfortunately, ANA had to advise the organisation that such monies would not be tax deductible, since ANA has as one of its aims, the advocacy and influencing of legislation. Since the tax deduction was a condition of the grant, the organisation withdrew the offer. At that same convention, the Board of Directors recommended that the House of Delegates authorise the incoming Board of Directors to take immediate action toward the development of a foundation similar to that of the American Hospital Association and the American Bar Association.

As a consequence, ANF was established in 1955 as a full-time co-ordinated program which is chartered for 'educational, scientific and charitable purposes,' and devoted to promoting and supporting nursing research and disseminating research findings. Currently, this is the only foundation in the country with the sole purpose of enhancing nursing research for the improvement of health care.

Structure of the Foundation

Nine members comprise the ANF Board of Trustees, several of whom must be ANA board members at the time of election to fulfill the legal requirements inherent in the ANA-ANF relationship. The full Board of Directors of ANA, sitting as members of ANF, elect the nine members to serve ANF. Subsequent to a re-evaluation and tightening of the foundation structure, the trustees decided to maintain a small core staff. ANF has three full-time employees - an administrative manager and two administrative assistants. The executive director, the controller, projects officer, and legal counsel are ANA staff and serve ANF through a contractual arrangement. Additional specific services are contracted from ANA as needed.

Financial Support

Through the years, funds for ANF have been solicited by fund raising letters and fund raising activities to potential foundations and corporate contributors. While foundations and corporate contributions help to support ANF, sustaining and major sources of funding have been generated from within the profession of nursing, with large contributions from ANA, the American Journal of Nursing Company, and individual nurses. In 1960, a national campaign for funds was initiated and continued until 1964, resulting in donations of over one-half million dollars for the foundation.

In 1978, using their investment portfolio as a basis, ANF established a permanent endowment fund, the principal of which has been restricted and cannot be used for operating purposes. In order to meet current and ever-increasing demands for foundation supported programs, and to enable long-range planning, the trustees believed a stable and strong financial base must be established. Toward that goal, the American Journal of Nursing Company, in April 1979, awarded a $100,000 challenge grant to ANF to match any monies received for endowment through December 31, 1981. More than $77,000 was contributed. Those funds were matched dollar for dollar by the American Journal of Nursing Company. Recognising that an endowment campaign is a long-term activity, the trustees initiated an annual 'giving' campaign conducted through direct mail solicitation. This direct mail campaign is designed to offer registered nurses the opportunity to contribute to the only existing national foundation with nursing research, demonstration projects, and scholarships as its priorities.

Programs of ANF
A primary goal of ANF is to encourage individuals, groups, and institutions to recognise and to utilise nursing's potential to improve health care in the United States. To accomplish this goal, ANF has had an intramural and extramural program, as well as arrangements for completion of research on a contractual basis between other organisations and ANF.

Extramural program. In the early years of ANF, grants were awarded for research to institutions having a similar tax-exempt status as ANF. Beginning in 1966, developmental grants for studies by individual nurses were awarded, and this program has continued yearly except for 1978 when fiscal considerations prohibited these awards. A major function of the individual grants is to encourage novice nurse researchers to develop skills before applying for support from major funding sources whose grants may average $100,000. Summary critiques are sent to all primary investigators submitting proposals to ANF for funding in order to provide constructive feedback and to encourage future investigation. Since the start of the program, a total of 147 grants have been awarded by the foundation, with a cost in excess of $900,000. These grants support studies of the work of nurses in general and private duty, psychiatric nursing, outpatient and industrial nursing, as well as student nurses. Subject areas include patient care, administration, education and clinical research.

In addition to individual grants, ANF contracted for completion of two projects. The first was a pilot project to survey the literature of nurses and patients in long-term care and the second was a project to study the informational needs of health professionals. The major emphasis of the latter project was to determine the ways in which abstracts collected by ANF's abstracting services were being used. Grants were also awarded to a hospital facility for the study of nursing in rehabilitation of elderly patients.

In addition to the above projects, the ANF board in 1963 granted a postdoctoral fellowship to a nurse scientist in the field of physiology who planned to develop nursing research in this field.

Intramural program. ANF has been instrumental in stimulating the conduct of research among nurses throughout the country. Beginning in 1960, consultant services on research were given collectively and individually in the field and at headquarters, a series of monographs of both extramural and intramural research was published, and a research abstracting service was undertaken with abstracts published in *Nursing Research*. Later, this abstracting service was discontinued by ANA. Staff of the foundation frequently attended and spoke at workshops, conventions, and meetings. Through the years, the following research, reports, and conferences contributed to the advancement of the profession in the area of research:

o   International Research Project. ANF was a medium for strengthening intercultural understanding and enriching world health services by maintaining contact with exchange nurses from abroad.
o   Hungarian Refugee Program. This program provided field services to nurses from Hungary making their home in the United States.
o   Report on the interaction of public health nurses and patients.
o   A study of family and patient adjustment to cardiac disease.
o   The upper New England research and education project for nurse practitioners on the utilisation of research findings in the improvement of patient care of the aged.
o   A study on the plan for indexing periodical literature of nursing. This study was crucial in proceeding with the development of the *International Nursing Index*. It was this study which encompassed the very real concerns of feasibility, cost, sponsorship, and support, and made it possible to reach a final decision regarding an index to nursing literature.
o   *Nursing Research Report* which was first published April 1966. Approximately 15,000 copies of this quarterly publication were distributed. It gave reports of studies conducted or supported by ANF. Information about ANF and its programs was also included

in the publication, which continued until December 1977.

o The first directory of nurses with earned doctorates was published in the September-October, 1969 issue of *Nursing Research*, with a listing of 504 nurses. Supplements in 1970 and in 1971 contained names of 677 nurses. After the 1972 edition, an international directory of nurses with earned doctorates was published in 1973 with a listing of 1,019 nurses from 20 countries. As an outgrowth of this work at ANF, the Cabinet on Nursing Research published a 1980 directory of nurses with earned doctorates in the United States, containing information on 1,964 nurses.

o The International Communications Network, which ANF helped develop in nursing, completed several major cooperative cross-cultural investigations and sponsored conferences and workshops.

o An interdisciplinary conference on nursing and health care administration.

The ANF also administers and raises funds for various activities of the American Academy of Nursing and for ANA projects. For example, ANF raised funds from corporations and foundations to support the Academy's second conference on the nursing role in primary care. In collaboration with the Academy, ANF received funds from the Robert Wood Johnson Foundation for two projects. The first was a workshop for nurses and physicians in practice and education within university health science centers to explore mutual responsibilities in patient care. The second was for the commissioning of papers that analysed future trends in nursing practice and the impact of such trends on education and employment. Other funds were obtained for preparation of a proposal for the development of a nursing taxonomy and for a presentation during the 1980 ANA convention on 'Health of Families in a Culture of Crisis'.

Two projects are, at present, administered by ANF. The Independence, Missouri Health Education Project (IM-HEP) is a program of health intervention, education, and screening for children in the Independence, Missouri school system. The Professional Practice for Nurse Administrators in Long-Term Care Facilities Project (NA-LTC) is jointly co-directed by project staff at ANF and staff of the American College of Nursing Home Administrators. This project seeks to improve care given to residents of long-term care facilities through professional development of nurse administrators in United States nursing homes.

The projects and research completed and continuing were possible by funding from several sources, notably the American Journal of Nursing Company, Rockefeller Foundation, Robert Wood Johnson Foundation, W.K. Kellogg Foundation, Bristol-Myers, Proctor and Gamble, Victor E. Speas Company, Heart Institute of the Public Health Service, U.S. Department of State, Center for Disease Control, Division of Nursing of the Public Health Service, and ANA, which also provides headquarters space and staff services.

Another means of supporting research is to make it visible. To this end, ANF planned a special achievement citations for research, the Distinguished Contribution to Nursing Science Award. It was first presented at the 1980 ANA convention, and the first recipient was Dr. Harriet H. Werley. In addition to a plaque to the recipient, a grant to a novice researcher is awarded in the recipient's name.

The foundation is continuing its 27-year tradition of supporting nursing research and working toward the recognition and the improvement of nursing practice.

AMERICAN ACADEMY OF NURSING (AAN)

The American Academy of Nursing is an organisation which allows significant opportunity for its members to contribute to the advancement of nursing and health care. It also provides for formal recognition and honor to individuals who are selected as fellows of the academy. The academy is seen

> ...as a working body which would operate in a climate in which current systems, ideas and practices may be challenged, new ideas in nursing and other fields explored, experimentation and innovation in nursing encouraged. The academy would share its ideas; it need not implement them. It would not duplicate functions of existing organisational units of ANA (ANA Convention Proceedings and Reports, 1970, p. 103).

The Academy is to work free from the constraints inherent in the work of ANA, where

solutions and action on immediate problems and
concerns of a diverse membership are demanded, yet
maintain ties with ANA.

Establishment of an Academy

At the 1958 convention, the ANA Committee on Current and Long-Term Goals presented two major goals
for future planning. The first goal concerned the
stimulation and encouragement of research and the
second was to 'establish ways within ANA to provide
formal recognition of personal achievement and
superior performance in nursing' (ANA Convention
Proceedings, 1958, p. 74). In line with this
second goal, a motion was passed at the 1964 convention 'that the ANA Board of Directors appoint a
committee to study and report at the biennial the
feasibility of and/or plan for the establishment of
an academy of nursing' (ANA Convention Proceedings,
1964, p. 33). Provisions for an academy to advance
knowledge, education, and nursing practice were
included in bylaws adopted by the 1966 House of
Delegates. With no certainty as to when and how
such a body would become a functioning reality, ANA
stated its intention to establish the academy of
nursing as a part of the professional association.
In January 1969, the ANA Board of Directors appointed an ad hoc committee to consider the concerns expressed by some members of the association
in regard to the proposed academy of nursing. This
ad hoc group met during 1969 and 1970 and discussed
the entrance of all original fellows. To plan for
the next steps toward establishment of the Academy,
a committee appointed by the ANA Board of Directors
met in March 1972, and reviewed the work of the ad
hoc committee, the reports and conclusions of the
groups that met during 1969 to resolve the issues
surrounding standards and certification, and the
recommendations for bylaw changes that were to go
to the 1972 ANA House of Delegates. The board
committee addressed itself: (a) to further clarification of the purposes and functions of an academy
of nursing; (b) to a plan for establishing the
Academy; (c) to criteria for selection of charter
fellows; and (d) to financing. Steps and target
dates for the establishment of the Academy were put
forth. Subsequently, 36 charter fellows of the
Academy were named by the ANA Board of Directors
following recommendations from ANA's cabinets and
divisions and from state nurses' associations. The
Academy became a reality on January 31, 1973.

At the first meeting of charter fellows on April 24, 1973, operating rules were adopted to establish and to elect fellows to a governing council, to clarify the role of this council, and to provide a sense of direction for the council's work. In September 1973, the charter fellows adopted by-laws for the Academy and operating rules for the Governing Council, including criteria for selection of future fellows of the Academy. The Academy was formed for the following purposes:

o to advance new concepts in nursing and health care;

o to identify and explore issues in health, in the professions, and in society as they affect and are affected by nurses and nursing;

o to examine the dynamics within nursing, inter-relationships among segments within nursing, and interaction among nurses as those factors affect the development of the nursing profession; and

o to identify and propose resolutions to issues and problems confronting nursing and health, including alternative plans for implementation (ANA House of Delegates Reports, 1978 - 1980, p. 173).

Structure of the Academy
The 36 charter fellows of the Academy elected ten members to a Governing Council who, in turn, elected a president, vice president, secretary, and treasurer from Governing Council members. ANA By-laws continued, in 1973, to provide that certification and endorsement by an ANA division on practice should be a necessary qualification for admission to the Academy. The action of the 1974 ANA House of Delegates removed this restriction from the bylaws, and cleared the way for the admission of additional fellows. It was intended that by 1976 and thereafter, academy membership should be composed of a proportionate distribution of nurse clinicians, educators, administrators, and researchers who have made a significant contribution to knowledge, education, nursing practice, or to the nursing profession in general. Fellows are selected by the membership committee and voted into the Academy by the total Academy membership.

Committees include a Priorities and Planning Committee, Finance Committee, Membership Committee, Scientific Sessions Committee, Public Relations Committee, Nominating Committee, Organizational Arrangements Committee, and various task forces with specific assignments.

Financial Support
The ANA Board of Directors allocated seed monies in an amount not exceeding $50,000 from the ANA reserve fund to cover the cost of establishing the Academy. Funds were used for consultation services and travel costs incidental to initiating the Academy. The ANA provides the necessary staff support, office space, equipment, services, and maintenance. It has also contributed over $65,000 over the last decade to the Academy.

The major portion of financing for the Academy derives from a series of recommendations from their Finance Committee in 1977 which were adopted by the Governing Council. These recommendations include: (a) a non-refundable application fee; (b) an initial year fee to new members; (c) an annual fee for membership; (d) opportunities for donations from members and contributions from others; (e) registration fees for self-supporting meetings and scientific sessions; (f) no honoraria or expenses paid for members participating in scientific sessions at annual meetings; and (g) receipt of income from publications. Support from grants to ANF for scientific sessions of the Academy have come from the Robert Wood Johnson Foundation, Alcoa Foundation, Monsanto Fund, C.V. Mosby Company, and Sterling Drug, Inc.

Programs and Publications of the Academy
In its short life, the Academy has accomplished many of the goals set forth in May 1972. In the years 1973 and 1974, fellows began to identify issues on which they would work. Considerable time and attention were also devoted to matters of organisation, by-laws, operating rules, criteria and procedures for selection of fellows, funding, and planning annual scientific sessions.

Annual scientific sessions and business meetings were begun in 1975 and have continued yearly. Proceedings of these sessions are published. New members of the Academy are welcomed and installed at the banquet held in conjunction with scientific sessions. In 1977, it was the decision of the

Governing Council to focus AAN annual scientific
sessions for a five-year period on nursing's influence on health care policy for the 1980s.

A Delphi survey of fellows of the Academy was
completed during the 1980 to 1982 biennium. The
purpose of the survey was to identify and priori-
tize those issues particularly susceptible to
impact by the Academy in keeping with its adopted
theme of nursing's influence on health care policy.
At the 1981 annual meeting, members concurred that
the primary focus of program activities over the
next ten years should be nursing's impact in the
health care delivery system. The Delphi survey
helped to identify specific issues to be addressed
in that regard. An initial assessment of the
results of the survey suggested that, at that time,
fellows saw the following as most critical and
susceptible to impact from Academy effort: (a)
public image of nursing; (b) reformulation of the
role of the nurse; and (c) research utilisation.
The scientific session on the public image of
nursing was held in 1982 and research utilisation
was the focus in 1983.

Three position statements have been issued by
the Academy concerning: (a) review of health care
services; (b) long-term care; and (c) nurses in
primary health care. Following the 1979 scientific
session, fellows adopted a resolution for the
unification of nursing service and nursing education.

In terms of publications, addresses presented
by the AAN presidents have been published in journals and/or distributed by the Academy. The following are examples of thought-provoking literature
published by the Academy:

o *Models for Health Care Delivery: Now and for
the Future* (The Academy, 1975).

o *Long-Term Care in Perspective: Past, Present
and Future Directions for Nursing* (The Academy, 1976).

o *Primary Care by Nurses: Sphere of Responsibility and Accountability* (The Academy, 1977).

o *Primary Care in a Pluralistic Society: Impediments in Health Care Delivery* (The Academy,
1978).

o *Nursing's Influence in Health Policy for the
Eighties* (The Academy, 1979).

o *Health Policy and Nursing Practice* (Aiken, 1981).

o *The Impact of Changing Resources on Health Policy* (Conway, 1981).

o *Priorities Within the Health Care System: A Delphi Survey* (Lindeman, 1981).

o *Nursing in the 1980s: Crises, Opportunities, Challenges* (Aiken and Gortner, 1982).

o *From Accommodation to Self-Determination: Nursing's Role in the Development of Health Care Policy* (Phillips, 1982).

Ongoing Activities
Current activities of the Academy are wide-ranging, and include the following endeavors:

o **Long-Term Care.** The task force on long-term care was established in 1980 to develop a proposal for a national demonstration project to upgrade care in long-term care facilities. The outcome of its work is the Teaching Nursing Home Project, cosponsored by the Robert Wood Johnson Foundation and the American Academy of Nursing. Members of the task force and other members of the Academy served on the advisory committee to the project, which made substantial grants to graduate programs in nursing that contracted to assume responsibility for nursing in long-term care facilities.

o **Hospice.** A task force was established in 1981 to plan and to identify funding for an Academy conference focused on hospice care. This special type of invitational conference was first held in 1983 with the stated purpose of discussing recent developments in hospice-type care, and implications for research and patient care practices.

o **Hospital Nursing Practice.** A task force on hospital nursing practice was established in early 1981 to examine the characteristics of systems impeding or facilitating professional nursing practice in hospitals. The task force embarked upon a project to examine characteristics of hospitals that function as 'magnets' for registered nurses. These are hospitals that consistently succeed in securing and retaining staff. The results of this project were published in 1983 (McClure, Poulin, Sovie & Wandelt).

o **Public Relations.** A task force on public relations was established in early 1981 to develop strategy (blueprint) as to how the Academy should proceed in improving the image of nursing. The task force recommended and the Governing Council approved the establish-ment of a series of media awards to be given by the Academy. One was presented at the AAN annual meeting in September 1981 to CBS News for the documentary, 'Nurse, Where Are You?'

o **Nursing Classics.** In 1983, a task force submitted for funding a proposal for a project designed to identify classic literary works in nursing, and to compile and analyse selected nursing classics in terms of professional, social, and political impact on society.

o **Faculty Practice.** In light of the 1979 reso-lution on unification of nursing service and nursing education, a proposal was prepared and submitted in April 1982 for a series of three annual symposia to identify, discuss, and promote nursing practice by faculty. The Robert Wood Johnson Foundation has funded the three symposia.

The American Academy of Nursing has had and will continue to have an impact on the nursing profession and on research activities.

CONCLUSIONS

The American Nurses' Association has accomplished the aims and goals it has set for itself in re-search. It has also collaborated with other nation-al organisations in areas of mutual concern regard-ing research and statistical data. To delineate all the various organisations and activities is beyond the scope of this paper; however, one group performs some co-ordinating functions. The Interagency Council on Nursing Statistics (ICONS), which began meeting regularly in 1956, has made a consistent effort to co-ordinate data and studies from several organisations, and to provide for greater communica-tion among organisations. This group has

representatives from governmental and major voluntary associations in the United States that gather
data on nursing and nurses. They meet twice yearly.
Several programs on data have been presented by
ICONS's members at ANA conventions.
Through various types of programs, ANA has been
involved internationally. Most prominent among
these is membership in the International Council of
Nurses (ICN) where ANA continues to promote collaborative efforts by nurses and others to meet health
needs throughout the world. Many visitors are
welcomed at ANA headquarters and are oriented to the
professional association and to nursing in the
United States.
The modified federation structure adopted by
the ANA House of Delegates July 1, 1982, makes the
interdependence of ANA and its constituents, state
nurses' associations, especially important. ANA
President, Eunice Cole, has stated:

> I believe that the new structure will enable us
> to identify more clearly which responsibilities
> are best carried out by ANA and which are best
> carried out by state associations. This will
> enable us to use our resources better. Roles
> and responsibilities more clearly defined,
> resources more appropriately used - to me that
> suggests that we are building an association
> that is strong and lean, ready to do its job
> well (Cole, *The American Nurse*, 1982).

The need to use resources appropriately may be
greatest in research where financial and human
assets are scarce. There is a tightening of funds
for research when the country's economic situation
is unstable, and there is still an insufficient
number of doctorally prepared nurses for the demands of nursing. Ways must be devised to identify
more clearly and differentiate research responsibilities at the state and national levels to
effectively use these scarce resources.
In a survey concerning state research groups
conducted in 1980 by the New York State Nurses
Association's Council on Research, 49 states and
three jurisdictions of the United States responded
(Frederickson, Oberst, Ventura, Schmitt, Noel, &
Corliss, in press). Eleven states had functioning
councils or commissions for research. Four states
reported no such groups, but stated that one was
needed or should be considered for the future, and
a state research group was neither functioning nor
planned by the remaining 37 states. To begin

discussion of responsibilities in research, the ANA Cabinet on Nursing Research conducted a program to promote information exchange and collaboration between ANA and state nurses' associations at the Council of Nurse Researchers' conference in 1983.

The inter-relationship between ANA, ANF, and AAN has been stressed. During the 1980 to 1982 biennium, officers and representatives of these three organisations met to assist in the articulation of the research aims and activities of the organisations. These meetings led to plans for the development of a Center for Research at ANA, the aim being to provide more effective and integrative use of financial and staff resources of the three organisations.

The purpose of the center is to provide an administrative unit which can co-ordinate the policy analysis, research, and statistical functions of the Research and Policy Analysis Department of ANA, ANF, and AAN. The objective of the center is to serve as a central mechanism for collection and analysis of information relevant to the nursing profession. If history is prologue, then ANA, ANF, and AAN combined for research effort in the ANA Center for Research creates optimism for greater research achievements in the future.

NOTES

1. The ANA House of Delegates adopted a modified federation structure at the ANA convention, July 1, 1982. State associations are now the members of ANA. Individual nurses hold membership in ANA through their membership in state associations. In reading this chapter, readers are reminded that former commissions are now called cabinets and the former Congress for Nursing Practice is a Cabinet on Nursing Practice.

REFERENCES

Aiken, L.H. (Ed.), (1981). American Academy of Nursing. *Health policy and nursing practice*. New York: McGraw-Hill.

Aiken, L.H., & Gortner, S.R. (Eds.), *American Academy of Nursing. Nursing in the 1980s: Crises, opportunities, challenges*. Philadelphia: J.B. Lippincott.

American Academy of Nursing (1975). *Models for health care delivery: Now and for the future.* Kansas City, MO: Author.

American Academy of Nursing (1976). *Long-term care in perspective: Past, present, and future directions for nursing.* Kansas City, MO: Author.

American Academy of Nursing (1977). *Primary care by nurses: Sphere of responsibility and accountability.* Kansas City, MO: Author.

American Academy of Nursing (1978). *Primary care in a pluralistic society: Impediments to health care delivery.* Kansas City, MO: Author.

American Academy of Nursing (1979). *Nursing's influence on health policy for the eighties.* Kansas City, MO: Author.

American Nurses' Association Convention Proceedings, House of Delegates and Sections (1958). New York: Author.

American Nurses' Association (1964) Proceedings, of the House of Delegates, Sections-Branches, Conference Groups (1964). New York: Author.

American Nurses' Association Proceedings and Reports (1970). New York: Author.

American Nurses' Association, Commission on Nursing Research (1975). *Human rights guidelines for nurses in clinical and other research.* Kansas City, MO: Author.

American Nurses' Association, Commission on Nursing Research (1976). *Research in nursing: Towards a science of health care.* Kansas City, MO: Author.

American Nurses' Association, Commission on Nursing Research (1979). *Nursing research: Synopsis of selected clinical studies.* Kansas City, MO: Author.

American Nurses' Association (1980). *Directory of nurses with doctoral degrees 1980.* Kansas City, MO: Author.

American Nurses' Association House of Delegates Reports, Report of the American Academy of Nursing (1978-1980, pp. 173-176). Kansas City, MO: Author.

American Nurses' Association (1981a). *Facts about nursing 80-81*. New York: American Journal of Nursing Company.

American Nurses' Association, Commission on Nursing Research (1981b). *Research priorities for the 1980s: Generating a scientific basis for nursing practice*. Kansas City, MO: Author.

American Nurses' Association, Commission on Nursing Research (1981c). *Guidelines for the investigative functions of nurses*. Kansas City, MO: Author.

Brimmer, P.F. (1978). Research and the American Nurses' Association. *Nursing Administration Quarterly, 2(4)*, 43-52.

Cole, E. (1982). Membership is still key to success under federation. *The American Nurse* editorial. *The American Nurse, 14(10)*.

Conway, M.E. (Ed.), (1981). American Academy of Nursing. *The impact of changing resources on health policy*. Kansas City, MO: American Nurses' Association.

Frederickson, K., Oberst, M.T., Ventura, M., Schmitt, M., Noel, N., & Corliss, I. (in press). Promoting nursing research through a state nurses' association.

Lindeman, C.A. (1981). American Academy of Nursing. *Priorities within the health care system: A delphi survey*. Kansas City, MO: American Nurses' Association.

McClure, M.L., Poulin, M.A., Sovie, M.D., & Wandelt, M.A. (1983). *Magnet hospitals*. Kansas City, MO: American Academy of Nursing.

Phillips, T.P. (Ed.), (1982). American Academy of Nursing. *From accommodation to self-determination: Nurses' role in the development of health care policy*. Kansas City, MO: American Nurses' Association.

Roth, A., Graham, D., & Schmittling, G. (1979). *1977 national sample survey of registered nurses, final report.* Kansas City, MO: American Nurses' Association.

Schulte, D.C. (1981). *Inventory of registered nurses 1977-1978.* Kansas City, MO: American Nurses' Association.

See, E.M. (1977). The ANA and research in nursing. *Nursing Research, 26(3),* 165-171.

CONTRIBUTORS

Ivo L. Abraham, RN, PhD
Assistant Professor, Frances Payne Bolton School of
Nursing, Case Western Reserve University
Cleveland, Ohio, USA

Moyra Allen, RN, PhD, DSc
Professor Emeritus
School of Nursing, McGill University
Montreal, Quebec, Canada

Pauline Brimmer, RN, PhD
Director, American Nurses' Association
Center for Nursing Research
Kansas City, Missouri, USA

M. Elizabeth Carnegie, RN, DPA
Editor Emeritus, *Nursing Research*; Distinguished
Visiting Lecturer, Hampton Institute School of
Nursing, and Independent Consultant
Hampton, Virginia, USA

Susan R. Gortner, MN, PhD, FAAN
Professor and Associate Dean for Research
School of Nursing
University of California, San Francisco
San Francisco, California, USA

Jack C. Hayward, BSc(Hon), PhD, SRN, RMN, RNT, DipN
Professor and Head, Department of Nursing Studies
Chelsea College, University of London
Chelsea, England

Lisbeth Hockey, OBE, PhD
International Consultant on Nursing Research, and
Formerly Director, Nursing Research Unit, Department
of Nursing Studies, The University of Edinburgh
Edinburgh, Scotland

Janet C. Kerr, RN, PhD
Professor and Associate Dean (Undergraduate Educa-
tion)
Faculty of Nursing
The University of Alberta
Edmonton, Alberta, Canada

Peggy Leatt, PhD
Associate Professor
Department of Health Administration
Community Health
Faculty of Medicine
University of Toronto
Toronto, Ontario, Canada

Sylvia R. Lelean, PhD, SRN, FRCN
Principal Nursing Officer (Research)
Department of Health and Social Security
London, England

Marian McGee, RN, DrPH
Associate Dean, Faculty of Health Sciences
Professor and Director, Nursing
University of Ottawa
Ottawa, Ontario, Canada

Janice M. Morse, RN, PhD (Nurs), PhD (Anthro)
Associate Professor, Faculty of Nursing
University of Alberta
Edmonton, Alberta, Canada

Shirley M. Stinson, RN, EdD, LLD
Associate Dean (Graduate Education and Research
Development), Faculty of Nursing, and Professor,
Faculty of Nursing and Department of Health Services
Administration and Medicine,
University of Alberta
Edmonton, Alberta, Canada

Mary Jane Ward, RN, PhD, FAAN
Associate Professor and Director of Research
School of Nursing
University of Colorado
Boulder, Colorado, USA

Valerie Wilmot, PhD
Senior Planning Officer
National Health Research and Development Program
Department of Health and Welfare
Government of Canada
Ottawa, Ontario, Canada

315